Active Older Adults:
Ideas for Action

Lynn Allen

Editor

With support from the
Sporting Goods Manufacturers Association (SGMA)

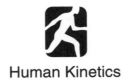

Human Kinetics

Library of Congress Cataloging-in-Publication Data

Active older adults : ideas for action / Lynn Allen, editor
 : with support from the Sporting Goods Manufacturers Association
(SGMA).
         p. cm.
     ISBN 0-7360-0128-X
     1. Physical fitness for the aged--United States. 2. Exercise for
the aged--United States. I. Allen, Lynn, 1958-   . II. Sporting
Goods Manufacturers Association (U.S.)
     GV482.6.A38   1999
     613.7'0446--DC21   98-35639
                                                         CIP

ISBN: 0-7360-0128-X

Acquisitions Editor: Judy Patterson Wright, PhD
Managing Editor: Cynthia McEntire
Assistant Editor: John Wentworth
Proofreader: Lisa Satterthwaite
Graphic Artists: Art Square and Francine Hamerski
Cover Designer: Jack Davis
Printer: United Graphics

Human Kinetics books are available at special discounts for bulk purchase. Special editions or book excerpts can also be created to specification. For details, contact the Special Sales Manager at Human Kinetics.

Printed in the United States of America   10 9 8 7
6 5 4 3 2 1

Human Kinetics
Web site: http://www.humankinetics.com

United States: Human Kinetics
P.O. Box 5076
Champaign, IL 61825-5076
1-800-747-4457
e-mail: humank@hkusa.com

Canada: Human Kinetics
475 Devonshire Road Unit 100
Windsor, ON N8Y 2L5
1-800-465-7301 (in Canada only)
e-mail: humank@hkcanada.com

Europe: Human Kinetics
P.O. Box IW14
Leeds LS16 6TR, United Kingdom
+44 (0) 113-278 1708
e-mail: humank@hkeurope.com

Australia: Human Kinetics
57A Price Avenue
Lower Mitcham, South Australia 5062
(08) 82771555
e-mail: humank@hkaustralia.com

New Zealand: Human Kinetics
P.O. Box 105-231, Auckland Central
09-523-3462
e-mail: humank@hknewz.com

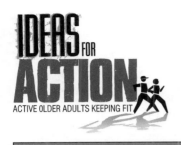

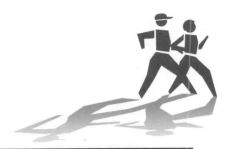

Contents

Part I
Program Ideas   1

Exercise Challenge   3

*Denise Horpedzhl -
Baton Rouge High School,
Baton Rouge, LA*

This activity involves the use
of an EXERCISE LOG to
track regular physical activity
over a 12-week period.
Acceptable activities are
listed for all age categories.
Includes participant letter,
activity list, and log sheet.

5 Plus 5   7

*Tim Lane & Sandi Ryan -
Iowa Department
of Public Health,
Des Moines, IA*

This community-based
program encourages
participants to EXERCISE
REGULARLY and make
WISE FOOD CHOICES.
An exercise log tracks
5 weekly exercise sessions
along with 5 daily servings
of fruits and vegetables.
Detailed sample worksheets
and handouts cover every
step of the process
necessary to administer
this program.

Line Dancing
for Seniors   51

*Donna Wilson & Jan Martin -
Leroy Springs
Recreation Complex,
Ft. Mills, SC*

This active, fun NO-COST
idea is easy to introduce to
a group of any size. Program
tips included.

Maple Knoll
Wellness Center   53

*Jan Montague -
Maple Knoll Village,
Cincinnati, OH*

The six DIMENSIONS OF
WELLNESS are identified
and examined. Includes
sample brochures and
handouts highlighting
various program offerings.

Walk Well 127

*Debbie Vold &
Susan Newville -
Hopkins Activity Center,
Hopkins, MN*
This exercise INCENTIVE
PROGRAM motivates
participants to get active
by following an imaginary
route and tracking miles
in a log book. Sample
materials are included.

Water Walking 133

*John R. Spannuth -
U.S. Water
Fitness Association,
Boynton Beach, FL*
This low impact, JOINT-
FRIENDLY EXERCISE
option is explained in
detail. Everything needed
to start up and administer
a program is included.

Young at Heart 141

*Kathy Kres -
Salem Athletic Club,
Salem, NH*
This is a program that is
conducted within a health
club. A list of ESSENTIAL
INGREDIENTS for staff and
safety considerations for
elder exercise are detailed
and explained. Class
descriptions and sample
handouts are included.

Part II
Resources 153

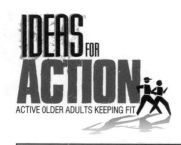

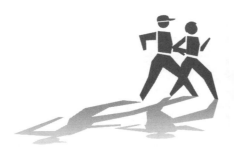

Introduction

If you didn't know your age, how old would you act?

Societal pressure tends to guide individuals of a certain age into specific patterns of thinking. The retirement mindset encourages one to "slow down" and "take it easy." Many individuals take these messages to heart, which can lead to destructive consequences.

The key finding of the Surgeon General's Report on Physical Activity and Health is that people **of all ages** can improve the quality of their lives through a lifelong practice of moderate physical activity.

FACT: The loss of strength and stamina attributed to aging is in part caused by reduced physical activity.

FACT: Activity decreases as we get older. By age 75, about one in three men and one in two women engage in no physical activity.

FACT: Social support from family and friends has been consistently and positively related to regular physical activity.

The purpose of this manual is to bring together a collection of fitness programming ideas for the older adult. A wide variety of ideas and activities from across the country are presented in this consistent, easy-to-implement format. Many of these programs have been nationally recognized for their contributions in the area of fitness programming for the older adult.

This manual will help solve the dilemma many activity directors working with older adults face… what do I do? Directions for implementing programming ideas are included, along with sample charts, brochures, newsletters and a listing of resources in order to insure the success of your program.

A common thread woven through all these successful fitness programs is the issue of social support found within each unique group. By learning how to weave this important thread into the activities of your participants, you will add vibrant color to the tapestry of their lives.

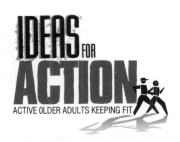

ACTIVE OLDER ADULTS KEEPING FIT

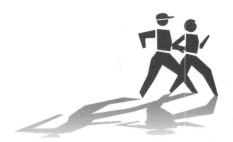

Tips for Promoting Your Fitness Program or Event

The following information can be applied to most any type of organization. The real key is planning. As they say, "planning is everything."

Promoting Through the Media

Developing a relationship with the media

One thing to understand about the media, whether it is newspaper, television or radio, is that the reporter or editor has priorities and deadlines. Know media deadlines and abide by them. A lot of other stories are after the same attention you are, and newspapers only have so much space, and radio and television stations only have so much air time they can dedicate to Public Service Announcements (PSAs).

The local newspaper will be your best bet for publicizing your fitness program or event. They care about what is happening in their community, and know their readers care, too.

Let's assume you have a press release written and you're ready to take it to the paper. **STOP** right there…did you make an appointment to see the editor? While many people take the route of "dropping off a press release," that's not the way to develop a relationship. Editors, reporters and anchor

people are very busy people, but don't think they aren't interested in what you have to say. In fact, they depend on people like you to bring them news. Just remember, by setting an appointment, you reduce the risk of barging in on someone who is trying to meet a deadline.

You may have to wait, and they may seem abrupt due to a pressing deadline you are unaware of, but be patient…and be helpful by bringing complete information…they'll ask for more, but try to make their job easy and you'll have a better chance of gaining their support. Make your presentation as specific as possible. Be sure to include facts as to why your program is interesting and be prepared to offer possible angles the story can be written from. Relate your event to current issues, if possible.

If you are mailing the press release, it will be worth your time to telephone each paper or station you're interested in and get the name of the editor, or news or program director who would be most interested. To make your job easier, type a list of media contacts and print labels in advance for easy and quick mailing. Time may pass before your information is published or aired, if at all. If considerable time has lapsed, follow up on your story and supply new or revised data concerning your program, thus keeping it "fresh."

Sometimes it may be necessary to contact the media by phone, such as when following up on the story. When contacting a morning paper by phone, your best bet is mid-to-late afternoon. Afternoon papers usually have deadlines around 11:00 a.m., so it's best to try after 11:30 a.m. or in the afternoon.

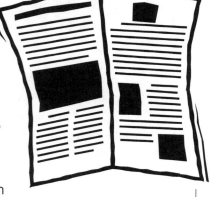

As a general rule, in developing important media relations, keep your contacts with media people active on a continuing basis. That doesn't mean become a pen pal or a nuisance on the phone. That will have an adverse affect on gaining their support. But a regular flow of news items and personal contact will enhance your chances of getting coverage for your program or event.

Quick Tips for Using Press Releases

- Get your release to the media in plenty of time before the event.

- Be professional...never try to get publicity by pressure or through business relationships or friendships.

- Don't ask when a story will appear.

- If you think your story would make a good feature story, rather than a straight news story, ask the editor about it...if it is worthy of space, the editor might assign the story and photographs.

- Attribute quotes to the highest ranking person in your organization.

- KITS can be put together when you have a release, photos, a program logo or program materials.

- PHOTOGRAPHS can be effective and are desired. Be sure the photos are clear and show people doing something which is relevant to your story.

  - 8 x 10" or 5 x 7" black and white glossy photos are preferred by newspapers

  - when possible, work with the newspaper photographer and set up each shot

  - try to limit the number of people in each shot to three unless you want a crowd shot

  - involve subjects in an activity; choose an interesting background but avoid clutter; provide props

  - identify all people and places in your photos; type the information on a gummed label or piece of paper and affix it to the back of photo and submit it with your press release.

Other Ideas for Publicizing Your Program or Event

- Radio or television talk shows.

- Consider cable television which offers 24-hour community news channels to publicize events and projects (contact the person in charge of local programming).

- Build displays or exhibits in shopping malls, banks, store windows, churches, recreation centers, utility companies, etc.; look professional.

- If you need community support, speak at local service club meetings.

- Develop posters; use talents of participants, art classes, art teachers, etc. Make posters colorful and creative. Hang them in offices, store windows, bowling alleys, churches, supermarkets, schools, libraries, bookstores, restaurants, etc.

- Create buttons and distribute to participants, planners, staff, etc.

- Send flyers home with participants.

Public Service Announcements (PSAs)

Both radio and television utilize Public Service Announcements, which are free to non-profit organizations. Here is basic information about PSAs.

- Contact the radio station 2-5 weeks in advance of when you want it to air.

- Approach area radio and television stations for taping local PSAs and creating artwork – use local personalities, participants or committee chairs in your PSAs.

- Send a thank you letter to the public service director and let him/her know the favorable comments and results you've received with the PSA.

Radio

Copy for radio is written differently than for print media, but you should still include the same facts: who, what, when, where, why and how.

Consider the format and audience of each radio station (top 40, country, news, etc.) and choose stations most suited to your message.

- Write in a conversational style.

- Spell out all numbers, etc., for reading.

- If you have difficult or unusual names or words, provide the phonetic pronunciations.

- Double or triple space copy.

- Use wide margins for editing.

- In upper left hand corner where you type your name and organization, include start and stop dates for airing as they pertain to your program or event. Also include the number of words in the PSA to help the program director gauge the reading time.

- To make sure your information is easy to read and understand, try reading copy aloud to someone else for their input.

Approximate PSA times for radio:
10 seconds (25 words of copy)
20 seconds (50 words of copy)
30 seconds (75 words of copy)
60 seconds (150 words of copy)

With radio you can also add music or sound effects; include voices from participants, etc. If you check with the public service director, they may produce a professional spot for you at no charge.

Television

This is a visual and audio medium, so write the copy in a conversational style for the announcer, and provide, if possible, a good photo or program logo for them to show on the television screen. Use art that is simple yet conveys your message. Ask for assistance from the station's art department if needed.

- Meet with the station's public service director to explain your ideas and find out what would be the best for promoting your organization.

- Television hits the highlights, so provide the most interesting and visual aspects of your unique program.

- Approximate PSA times for television:

  10 seconds (25 words of copy) 20 seconds (45 words of copy) 30 seconds (65 words of copy) 60 seconds (125 words of copy)

You'll find the number of words for television is less than for radio because television copy is read slower.

Open House

An excellent way to showcase your fitness program is by hosting an open house or special event.

This enables prospective participants to meet program leaders. It provides an opportunity for local media coverage, a tour of your facility, as well as time to "prime the pump" for sign-up.

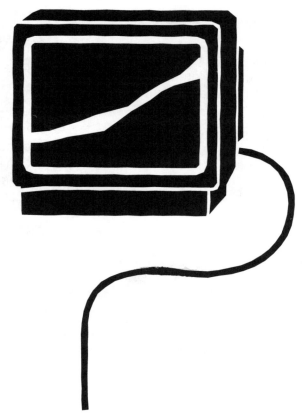

```
Your Name
Title
Organization
Address
City/State/Zip
Phone                                    FOR IMMEDIATE RELEASE


            GUIDELINES FOR WRITING PRESS RELEASES

YOUR TOWN, State- Suggestions for preparing and placing a news
release or PR release are being outlined here for individuals
to read and use as guidelines when promoting their fitness program
and related activities.

      Releases should be typed and photocopied cleanly on white
8 1/2" x 11" paper. Mail them first class to the media in your
area, including radio and television news directors and local
newspapers. It's best to deliver a copy personally to city editors
of local newspapers.

      Other guidelines:

      IDENTIFICATION: The name, organization, address and telephone
number of the person to contact for more information should appear
at upper left.

      RELEASE DATE: Your release should be "immediate,"
unless you are submitting the news release prior to an event (for
publication immediately after the event), use a hold release and be
specific: FOR RELEASE AFTER 8:00 P.M. WEDNESDAY, MAY 20, 1998.

      SPACING: Use wide margins, 1 1/2 inches, so editors can write
in them, AND double space so editors can edit the story.


                          -more-
```

Release Guidelines 2

HEADLINES: Write an eye-catching headline that is to the point. Some editors will rewrite the headline. Leave about 2 inches between release line and body of copy so editor can insert or rewrite the headline. If you do include a headline, type it in all capital letters and center it.

SUMMARY LEAD: In the first paragraph, try to include the who, what, when, where type of information. Editors expect the most important information to be at the beginning and will often start cutting copy from the bottom up. Use a lead that will catch and hold a busy reader's attention. Use short, punchy sentences.

LENGTH: If it is a news release, keep it to one or two pages-features two to three. Edit your material to bare facts and make sure it is accurate, timely and newsworthy. Do not split a paragraph between the first and second page. When you get to an inch from the bottom of the page and still have more copy, center the word "-more-" to indicate the story continues. At the top left of the second sheet, type a 2 or 3 word description of article and page number.

ACCURACY: Make sure spelling and grammar are 100% accurate. Proofread very carefully. Double check your facts.

PLACEMENT: Take your press release to local newspapers, television and radio stations. Discuss special news with specialized writers. Never take the same story twice to the same place.

At the end of your release, center the editorial symbol for "the end" which is either -30- or ### at the bottom of the page.

###

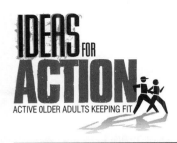

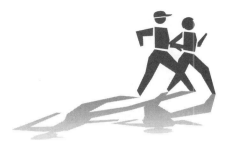

Physical Activity and Health
for Older Adults

Key Messages

- Older adults, both male and female, can benefit from regular physical activity.

- Physical activity need not be strenuous to achieve health benefits.

- Older adults can obtain significant health benefits with a moderate amount of physical activity, preferably daily. A moderate amount of activity can be obtained in longer sessions of moderately intense activities (such as walking) or in shorter sessions of more vigorous activities (such as fast walking or stairwalking).

- Additional health benefits can be gained through greater amounts of physical activity, either by increasing the duration, intensity or frequency. Because risk of injury increases at high levels of physical activity, care should be taken not to engage in excessive amounts of activity.

- Previously sedentary older adults who begin physical activity programs should start with short intervals of moderate physical activity (5-10 minutes) and gradually build up to the desired amount.

- Older adults should consult with a physician before beginning a new physical activity program.

- In addition to cardiorespiratory endurance (aerobic) activity, older adults can benefit from muscle-strengthening activities. Stronger muscles help reduce the risk of falling and improve the ability to perform the routine tasks of daily life.

Facts

- The loss of strength and stamina attributed to aging is in part caused by reduced physical activity.

- Inactivity increases with age. By age 75, about one in three men and one in two women engage in no physical activity.

- Among adults aged 65 years and older, walking and gardening or yard work are, by far, the most popular physical activities.

- Social support from family and friends has been consistently and positively related to regular physical activity.

Benefits of Physical Activity

- Helps maintain the ability to live independently and reduces the risk of falling and fracturing bones.

- Reduces the risk of dying from coronary heart disease and of developing high blood pressure, colon cancer, and diabetes.

- Can help reduce blood pressure in some people with hypertension.

- Helps people with chronic, disabling conditions improve their stamina and muscle strength.

- Reduces symptoms of anxiety and depression and fosters improvements in mood and feelings of well-being.

- Helps maintain healthy bones, muscles and joints.

- Helps control joint swelling and pain associated with arthritis.

What Communities Can Do

- Provide community-based physical activity programs that offer aerobic, strengthening and flexibility components specifically designed for older adults.

- Encourage malls and other indoor or protected locations to provide safe places for walking in any weather.

- Ensure that facilities for physical activity accommodate and encourage participation by older adults.

- Provide transportation for older adults to parks or facilities that provide physical activity programs.

- Encourage health care providers to talk routinely to their older adult patients about incorporating physical activity into their lives.

- Plan community activities that include opportunities for older adults to be physically active.

For more information, contact:

Centers for Disease Control and Prevention
National Center for Chronic Disease Prevention and Health Promotion
Division of Nutrition and Physical Activity, MS K-46
4770 Buford Highway, NE
Atlanta, GA 30341-3724
Phone: 1-888-CDC-4NRG
   or 1-888-232-4674 (Toll Free)
Web-Site: http://www.cdc.gov

The President's Council on Physical Fitness and Sports
200 Independence Avenue SW
HHH Building, Room 738H
Washington, DC 20201
Phone: (202) 690-9000
Fax: (202) 690-5211
Web-Site:
www.os.dhhs.gov/progorg/ophs/pcpfs.htm

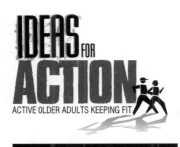

IDEAS FOR ACTION
ACTIVE OLDER ADULTS KEEPING FIT

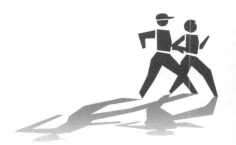

Part I

Program Ideas

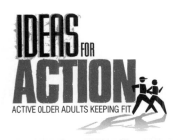

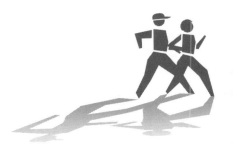

ACTIVE OLDER ADULTS KEEPING FIT

PROGRAM:

Exercise Challenge

Organization: Baton Rouge High School
2825 Government Street
Baton Rouge, LA 70806
Phone: (504) 383-0520
Fax: (504) 344-3066
Contributor: Denise Horpedzhl

Program Objectives

• to promote regular physical activity

• to encourage individuals of all ages to increase their activity level

Materials/Equipment Needed

• depends on the activity/activities chosen from the list

Procedures and Teaching Strategies

• use goals and rewards to encourage regular physical activity over a 12-week period

• encourage participation of all ages

• urge participants to exercise in groups as added motivation

Program Description

This activity involves the use of an EXERCISE LOG to track regular physical activity over a 12-week period.

Each week has 42 boxes and each box represents five (5) minutes of exercise. For each five (5) minutes of exercise, shade in one (1) box. Acceptable exercise activities

are listed on the following page. Activities are listed for a variety of ages to encourage multi-generational involvement. At the end of the 12-week program, all boxes should be filled in. The completed log can then be exchanged for an EXERCISE CHALLENGE T-shirt.

Program Tips

Awards such as T-shirts and printed certificates may be funded by a donation from a local company.

Program graphic to be used on T-shirts and promotional materials could be determined through an art contest.

Encourage the buddy system. Have participants team up with one another to keep each other motivated.

Plan an awards ceremony to distribute the T-shirts earned during the EXERCISE CHALLENGE. Make note of individual accomplishments made during this 12-week session. Challenge participants to continue "the exercise habit" with new and bigger goals.

Publicize the program to the local media.

Acceptable Activities

Children (Up to age 8)	Youth, Teens, Adults (Ages 9 - 55)	Older Adults* (Over 55)
soccer	aerobic dancing	gardening
tennis	hiking	painting (walls)
walking	walking/jogging	changing a tire
jogging	running	raking leaves
bike riding	circuit weight training	sweeping driveway
jump rope	skiing (water/snow)	stairclimbing
swimming	golf	washing car/boat
basketball	handball	table tennis
rollerskating	racquetball	shuffleboard
	rollerskating	all Senior Olympic activities
	rowing	
	soccer	
	basketball	* In addition to all activities listed for other groups
	tennis	
	softball	
	stairclimbing (machine)	
	treadmill	
	swimming	

Dear EXERCISE CHALLENGE Participant:

A survey has shown that 90% of all Americans believe that participation in some kind of regular physical activity is important. Many are now realizing the value of being active and feeling fit no mater what their age. However, many people, both young and old, are not as physically fit as they should be.

Many people do only the least amount of exercise possible. Studies have shown that fitness declines with age. This lack of fitness is the result of our inactive lifestyle that depends on the car, television and other machines. You probably do not need a high level of fitness to live in a world that uses many machines, but regular physical activity is necessary if your body is to function properly. That is why it is important to follow a regular exercise program.

Fitness For Life
Corbin and Lindsey

ACCEPTABLE ACTIVITIES

Children	**Youth, Teens, Adults**	**Older Adults***
(Up to age 8)	(Ages 9 - 55)	(Over 55)
soccer	aerobic dancing	gardening
tennis	hiking	painting (walls)
walking	walking/jogging	changing a tire
jogging	running	raking leaves
bike riding	circuit weight training	sweeping driveway
jump rope	skiing (water/snow)	stairclimbing
swimming	golf	washing car/boat
basketball	handball	table tennis
rollerskating	racquetball	shuffleboard
	rollerskating	all Senior Olympic activities
	rowing	
	soccer	* In addition to all activities
	basketball	listed for other groups
	tennis	
	softball	
	stairclimbing (machine)	
	treadmill	
	swimming	

NAME _____

ADDRESS _____

TELEPHONE _____

T-shirt size (circle one) 　XXL 　　XL 　　L 　　M 　　S 　　14-16 　　10-12

TIP: When reproducing for handouts, copy pages 5 and 6 back to back.

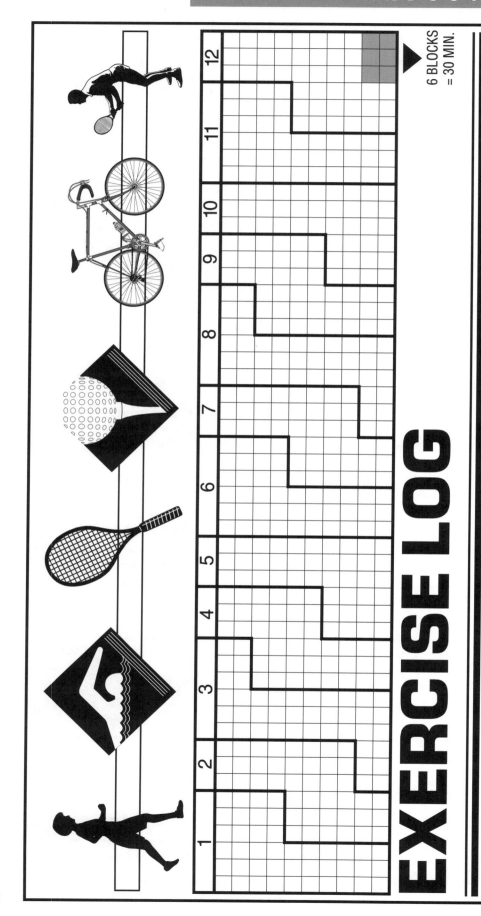

▶ 6 BLOCKS = 30 MIN.

EXERCISE LOG

DIRECTIONS:

★ This EXERCISE LOG is divided into 12 weeks. Each week has 42 boxes and each box represents 5 minutes of exercise. For each 5 minutes of exercise shade in 1 box. If you walk for 30 minutes, shade in 6 boxes. (Use only whole boxes when shading in minutes.) ★ At the end of the 12-week program, all boxes should be filled in. Return your log to _____ along with $ _____ and you will receive a T-shirt with the EXERCISE CHALLENGE logo on it. You may choose to do this every 12 weeks, however T-shirts are given only once.

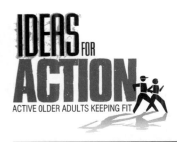

ACTIVE OLDER ADULTS KEEPING FIT

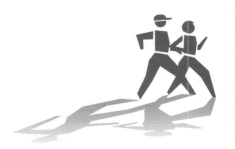

5 Plus 5

Organization:	Iowa Department of Public Health
	Bureau of Health Promotion
	Lucas State Office Building, Third Floor
	321 East 12th Street
	Des Moines, IA 50319-0075
Phone:	(515) 281-7833
Fax:	(515) 281-4535
e-mail:	tlane@idph.state.ia.us
Web-Site:	idph.state.ia.us/sa/hprom.htm
Contributors:	Tim Lane and Sandi Ryan

Some information in the **5 Plus 5** Program was adapted from previous efforts by state health agencies in Minnesota, New York and California. In Iowa, the Story County **5 Plus 5** Challenge Committee continued the development process with their participant materials.

The **5 Plus 5** message is based on the following recommendations.

5 A Week: The Surgeon General's Report on Physical Activity and Health states everyone should accumulate 30 minutes or more of moderate physical activity most days of the week. Thus, *5 A Week*.

5 A Day: The National Cancer Institute and the Produce for Better Health Foundation state everyone should eat at least five servings of fruits and vegetables each day as part of a high-fiber, low-fat diet. Thus, *5 A Day*.

Older adults were just one of the many groups targeted for involvement in this program. Whether you involve the total

community in your program planning or focus on just the older adult population, the **5 Plus 5** program is an exciting opportunity to increase the health and fitness of your community.

Program Objectives

- to encourage participants to be physically active for 30 minutes at least five (5) days a week

- to encourage participants to eat five (5) servings of fruits and vegetables every day as part of a high-fiber, low-fat diet

Program Description

Community-based programs to increase physical activity or improve nutrition offer tremendous health benefits. Integrating physical activity and nutrition programs creates a synergistic effect which leads to increased fitness and reduced risks for heart disease, certain cancers, stroke, diabetes mellitus, obesity and related chronic diseases.

The circumstances surrounding the creation of a **5 Plus 5** physical activity/nutrition program will vary among organizations. Regardless of the size of the community or the group's financial resources, the step-by-step approach outlined here will provide the information and support required to design, implement, and evaluate a community-based physical activity/nutrition program.

A 9-Step Process

Use the following nine steps to plan, implement, evaluate and sustain the physical activity/nutrition program.

1. Select a Coordinator and Core Planning Group

Begin by identifying a project coordinator. The coordinator should appoint a core group of three to six people to assist in program planning.

2. Develop a Community Profile

Developing a community profile will help the core planning group identify target population(s), effective intervention strategies, and potential community partners. The profile should include the following items.

- Geographic information

- Demographic attributes

- Epidemiological information

- Community resources

- Key community leaders

Geographic Information: Get to know the geographical layout of your service area. Map key sites, such as schools, churches, grocery stores, and other places where participants can meet for exercise and to buy food.

Demographic Attributes: Define the key characteristics of the community's various population groups. Include demographic attributes such as age, sex, ethnicity, income and educational level. (The U.S. Census Bureau is the most comprehensive source of this type of information.)

Epidemiological Information: Information on the health habits, morbidity (disease) and mortality (death) rates for your area may be available from the National Center for Health Statistics (NCHS) of the U.S. Department of Health and Human Services (301/436-8500). (See WORKSHEET 1 for help in analyzing and prioritizing the demographic and epidemiological data gathered.)

Community Resources: Develop a list of possible potential partners of the physical activity/nutrition program. The list should include government units, schools, churches, civic groups, public and private health agencies and facilities, major businesses and industries, media and emergency services. (See WORKSHEET 2 to create a listing.)

Key Community Leaders: It is important to identify the "movers and shakers" in your community. (See WORKSHEET 3 and 4.) This information will help provide

- important clues about how to launch the project;

- an idea of the level of community awareness about physical activity and nutrition needs; and

- an indication of the level of support for the project, as well as identifying potential project partners.

3. Establish a Community Advisory Board or Coalition

Coalitions can

- use limited community resources efficiently;

- provide more skills than a single organization;

- build trust among community organizations;
- help to ensure that community interventions and materials are culturally sensitive;
- prevent duplication of efforts and competition among community organizations for limited resources; and
- convey a powerful message about the importance of physical activity/nutrition programs to the community.

You can select members of the coalition from among the opinion leaders identified in the survey. In addition, consider using members of organizations such as County Extension Service; Parks and Recreation Department; community schools, local nutrition/health/wellness coalition; YMCA/YWCA/JCC; local media; service organizations and local voluntary agencies.

4. Conduct a Community Inventory Survey

Before beginning the program, it is important to know what community programs and activities already address these issues. Gather this information by completing a community resource inventory. (See WORKSHEET 5.) This will help to

- identify existing physical activity/nutrition programs in the community;
- identify gaps in current programming;
- identify potential partners for the program; and
- learn about the potential for coordinating the program with an existing one. (See WORKSHEET 6.)

5. Identify Priorities and Appropriate Activities

Based upon the information gathered in the community profile and the community resource inventory, your organization can set realistic goals for the program. Use WORKSHEET 7 at a brainstorming session to choose program activities. WORKSHEET 8 can help a group decide if an activity is feasible.

6. Develop a Plan

Having identified community physical activity/nutrition needs, target groups, media and activities, the next step is to develop the program plan. What are you going to do and how are you going to do it? Compile a task chart, listing all the steps needed to conduct each activity. Provide regular updates to all program partners.

7. Promote! Promote! Promote!

Deciding how to promote the program over a course of time will increase the likelihood of the program's success. WORKSHEET 7 will assist in planning the promotion. Remember to include other events, such as a fun run or walk held before or after the event, state and national campaigns, and national health promotion observances.

8. Evaluate the Effort

Evaluating the program's progress and outcomes helps determine which strategies or tasks worked well, and directions for the future.

9. Sustain the Momentum

Often after large community-wide efforts, the temptation is to fall into a lull for a period of time. A more effective strategy is to use the time at the conclusion of a program to debrief and identify what worked, what didn't, and why.

Remember to take time to recognize and thank volunteers and community groups who made the program(s) possible. There are many ways to say thank you, including paid advertisements, direct mail pieces, a letter to the editor, personal notes, or a party.

WORKSHEET 1

ANALYZING COMMUNITY DATA

1. Describe the physical activity/nutrition-related health problems in your community.

Notes:

Health Problems	Relation to Physical Activity	Relation to Nutrition

2. Who are the potential target audiences for your physical activity/nutrition program? What are the age, sex, ethnicity, places of work, income, and residence of target audiences?

Notes:

Target Audience	Age	Sex	Ethnicity	Workplace	Income Levels	Residence

3. What are some of the factors in the community that influence physical activity/ nutrition-related health problems, i.e., availability of exercise facilities, number of grocery stores with labeling programs, number of restaurants, availability of public health nutrition programs, etc.?

Notes:

Community Factor	How Widely Available	To What Population(s) is it Available

WORKSHEET 2A

LIST OF ORGANIZATIONS

Note: Before starting, you may want to check with other organizations to see if they have already completed a resource inventory. Ask if they are willing to share it.

Health
(voluntary health organizations, county medical societies, hospitals, health departments, social services)

Organization	Phone Number

Business and Industry
(worksites, restaurants, business coalitions, unions, chambers of commerce)

Organization	Phone Number

Political and Legal Groups
(city council, county supervisors, health boards, bar associations, law enforcement agencies)

Organization	Phone Number

WORKSHEET 2B

LIST OF ORGANIZATIONS

Education
(schools, teacher groups, parent groups, colleges, adult education)

Organization	Phone Number

Media
(newspapers, radio, television)

Organization	Phone Number

Information
(libraries)

Organization	Phone Number

Recreation
(recreation departments, YMCA/YWCA/JCC, health clubs, school athletic departments)

Organization	Phone Number

Community Groups
(service clubs, religious organizations, citizen action groups, civic groups)

Organization	Phone Number

WORKSHEET 3

IDENTIFYING OPINION LEADERS

Start the process by asking a known, influential leader (see paragraph titled *Key Community Leaders* on page 8), such as a banker, director of the chamber of commerce, or a newspaper editor one of the sample questions. Next, interview one of the persons he/she names in the same manner until those named most often (perhaps three or more times) are in turn interviewed. This process can continue until the interviewer can largely predict the interviewee's responses.

Sample questions

Would you please name six or eight persons who you think have the most influence in general community affairs in (name the community)?

Which persons in this community carry the most weight in community affairs?

Which locally powerful people can get things done or can stop local projects?

Whose approval is usually needed to get people in this community to accept or reject important change?

Identifying leaders in special areas or minority groups

Would you please name two or three persons who have the most influence in each of the following areas (or groups)?

An approach to identifying influential groups is to ask

Would you please name the groups or organizations having the most influence on general community affairs in this community?

Or to be more specific in the area of health:

Which organization or group in this community do you think would be influential in determining whether or not a program to improve the health of community residents could be successful?

WORKSHEET 4A

COMMUNITY OPINION SURVEY

Identified leaders should be sent a letter describing your coalition or organization and stating that you'll be calling to set up an interview appointment.

Name:

_____

Title:

_____

Address:

_____

Phone:

_____

Date of Interview:

_____

1. In your opinion, what factors contribute to the high rate of sedentary lifestyle and poor nutrition in (your community)?

2. What do you think should be done to more effectively address physical activity patterns and nutrition in this area?

3. What barriers, if any, do you see to implementing a project to address sedentary lifestyle and poor nutrition in the community? (If none are identified, skip to question 5.)

WORKSHEET 4B

COMMUNITY OPINION SURVEY

4. What strategies would you suggest for overcoming these barriers?

5. What role could you play to help us implement physical activity/nutrition projects in our community? (Do not read out the choices below. Use them as suggestions and as a guide for recording responses.)

☐ Serve on a coalition
☐ Serve on a task force or committee
☐ Public endorsement/testimonial

☐ Appoint a person to work on the project
☐ Donate resources, i.e., meeting space, advertising, personnel, funds, etc.

6. Could you suggest a contact person in other organizations/groups in our community who could take part in physical activity/nutrition projects?

7. Who in our community would you consider critical to the success of physical activity/nutrition projects?

8. Are there any other suggestions or ideas that you can give me as we prepare to get physical activity/nutrition projects started?

9. Are there any questions you would like to ask me?

Thank you for your time and support. I'll be in touch with you again to let you know how the project is progressing and how you can best help to insure the project's success.

Adapted from the Florence Heart to Heart Program, South Carolina Cardiovascular Disease Prevention

WORKSHEET 4C

COMMUNITY OPINION SURVEY

Demographics of the Leaders

Note: Keep records of the leaders you interview to insure that you are getting input from different segments of the community. Try to record this demographic information on the respondents, without directly asking the questions. This information should be kept confidential and should not be attached to the survey or the final report.

Sex: ☐ Female ☐ Male

Race/Ethnicity: ☐ White ☐ African American ☐ Hispanic

☐ Native American ☐ Asian ☐ Other

Age: ☐ <18 ☐ 18-24 ☐ 25-44 ☐ 45-64 ☐ 65+

Affiliation that resulted in respondent being selected for survey:

☐ Business Person ☐ City/County Official

☐ Civic Association Member ☐ Clergy/Church Leader

☐ Health Professional ☐ Law Enforcement Official

☐ Local Celebrity ☐ Media Representative

☐ Neighborhood Leader ☐ School Board Member/ Administrator/Educator

☐ Social Services Provider ☐ Other

☐ Youth Peer Leader

How long has the respondent been a member of the community?

☐ <3 years ☐ 3-10 years ☐ >10 years

In what town/neighborhood/school district/etc. does the respondent live?

WORKSHEET 5A

SURVEY OF COMMUNITY ACTIVITIES

This survey lists some questions you might want to ask an organization. Because some organizations may feel threatened by your questions and wonder about your motives, review with them your reasons for conducting this survey. Offer to share the results with them and other community organizations. Depending upon the objectives of your group, you may add or delete questions.

Organization:

_____

Name of contact person:

_____

Address: _____ Phone: _____

_____

Type of organization:

_____

Target populations served by the organization:

_____

1.   Did you provide any lectures/classes on physical activity/nutrition last year?

2.   How many classes/lectures?

3.   Fees for the classes?

4.   How many people participated?

5.   Where are the classes/lectures held?

WORKSHEET 5B

SURVEY OF COMMUNITY ACTIVITIES

6. Did you offer any screening or assessment programs? How many people participated?

7. Did you provide any special events or promotional activities?

8. Did another organization co-sponsor any of your classes or special events?

9. Do you make any print materials or videos regarding physical activity/nutrition available to the public? Do you charge a fee?

10. Which classes/programs do you plan to continue?

11. What new classes/programs do you plan to offer in the next year?

12. Do you believe the methods you've used for reaching your target audience have been successful? If not, how do you plan to change?

WORKSHEET 6A

SUMMARY OF CURRENT ACTIVITIES

SETTING			
STRATEGY	**Schools**	**Worksites**	**Health Care**
AWARENESS: Increase level of awareness or interest in the topic, i.e., newsletters, posters, health fairs, health screenings, media. **LIFESTYLE:** Change the behavior of the individual, i.e., behavior modification, experiential learning and skill building activities. **SUPPORTIVE ENVIRONMENT:** Programs that change the environment or encourage healthy habits and discourage unhealthy ones, i.e., marked walking trails, nutrition labeling of restaurant menus.			

Notes:

WORKSHEET 6B

SUMMARY OF CURRENT ACTIVITIES

SETTING			
Restaurants	**Grocery**	**Community**	**STRATEGY**
			AWARENESS: Increase level of awareness or interest in the topic, i.e., newsletters, posters, health fairs, health screenings, media. **LIFESTYLE:** Change the behavior of the individual, i.e., behavior modification, experiential learning and skill building activities. **SUPPORTIVE ENVIRONMENT:** Programs that change the environment or encourage healthy habits and discourage unhealthy ones, i.e., marked walking trails, nutrition labeling of restaurant menus.

Notes:

WORKSHEET 7A

INVENTORY OF POTENTIAL ACTIVITIES

SETTING			
STRATEGY	**Schools**	**Worksites**	**Health Care**
AWARENESS: Increase level of awareness or interest in the topic, i.e., newsletters, posters, health fairs, health screenings, media.			
LIFESTYLE: Change the behavior of the individual, i.e., behavior modification, experiential learning and skill building activities.			
SUPPORTIVE ENVIRONMENT: Programs that change the environment or encourage healthy habits and discourage unhealthy ones.			

Notes:

WORKSHEET 7B

INVENTORY OF POTENTIAL ACTIVITIES

SETTING			
Restaurants	**Grocery**	**Community**	**STRATEGY**
			AWARENESS: Increase level of awareness or interest in the topic, i.e., newsletters, posters, health fairs, health screenings, media. **LIFESTYLE:** Change the behavior of the individual, i.e., behavior modification, experiential learning and skill building activities. **SUPPORTIVE ENVIRONMENT:** Programs that change the environment or encourage healthy habits and discourage unhealthy ones.

Notes:

WORKSHEET 8

IS THE PROGRAM RIGHT FOR US?

If you are developing your own program or are adapting an existing program, there are points to consider before implementing it. Use this worksheet for each activity to determine if the program is really right for your organization and community. Give the activity one point for each criterion it meets. The first four criteria are required. You might want to have program partners fill the worksheet out together. When completed, determine if the number of problems you will have will jeopardize the successful implementation of the program.

Can be accomplished in the given time period.

Can be accomplished within the given budget.

Is wanted by the target population.

Is needed by the target population.

Fits with the goals of our organization and partners.

Does not duplicate an existing community program.

Will be feasible to implement.

Other organizations may be willing to collaborate.

Has the potential to become incorporated into the community.

The organization has the expertise (or access to expertise) to develop and implement the program.

Can be evaluated.

THE PHYSICAL FIVE: PHYSICAL ACTIVITY PROGRAM STRATEGIES

A New Message for the '90s – Moderate Physical Activity

According to the Surgeon General's Report on Physical Activity and Health, inactivity is a serious, nationwide problem. Its scope poses a challenge to public health for reducing the national burden of unnecessary illness and premature death.

Regular physical activity, performed on most days of the week, reduces the risk of developing or dying from some of the leading causes of illness and death in the United States. It also improves health in the following ways:

- reduces the risk of dying prematurely;
- reduces the risk of dying from heart disease;
- reduces the risk of developing diabetes;
- reduces the risk of developing high blood pressure;
- helps reduce blood pressure in people who already have high blood pressure;
- reduces the risk of developing colon cancer;
- reduces feelings of depression and anxiety;
- helps control weight;
- helps build and maintain healthy bones, muscles, and joints;
- helps older adults become stronger and better able to move about without falling; and
- promotes psychological well being.

Recommendations

1. Everyone should accumulate 30 minutes or more of moderate physical activity most days of the week. This program features **5 A Week** to simplify the message. The message coincides with the national **5 A Day** nutritional program which balances the **5 Plus 5** approach.

Scheduling more activity into the daily routine is an effective way to improve health. Activities that can contribute to the 30-minute total include climbing stairs instead of using the elevator, gardening, raking leaves, dancing and walking. The recommended 30 minutes of physical activity may also come from planned activity or recreation such as jogging, playing tennis, swimming and cycling.

2. Most adult Americans fail to meet this recommended level of moderate physical activity.

Persons who currently do not engage in regular physical activity should begin by incorporating a few minutes of increased activity into their day, building up gradually to 30 minutes of additional physical activity. Those who are irregularly active should strive to adopt a more consistent pattern of activity. Regular participation in physical activities that develop and maintain muscular strength and joint flexibility are also recommended.

Adults beginning a new physical activity program should check with their doctors. This is an especially important recommendation for adults who have been sedentary for a number of years.

Never Too Late

No one is too old to enjoy the benefits of regular physical activity. Evidence shows that muscle-strengthening exercises can reduce the risk of falling and fracturing bones and can improve the ability to live independently.

Program Models

Successful physical activity programs are a combination of planning, insight, support, personalities and sometimes luck.

Recruitment

How do you recruit sedentary adults to join your program? Here are a few tips based on the experience of program leaders and research on successful physical activity programs.

Know Your Audience: A program is more likely to be successful if it is designed for a specific audience. Before you begin, talk informally to members of your target group. Ask their interest in a physical activity program, reasons they are or are not active, their ideas for a new program and their willingness to be involved.

Use Community Members to Recruit New Participants: Word of mouth is the most powerful recommendation of a good program. If you are starting a **5 Plus 5** program, consider training members of your target audience as walking club leaders. Ask community members to recruit their friends, fellow employees and family to join the program.

Emphasize the Benefits of Physical Activity: Many people believe they need to jog or engage in other strenuous activity in order to gain any health benefits from exercise. New research suggests that regular activity is what counts. For the inactive, even light to moderate physical activity can improve health. This positive message appeals to many who may not otherwise participate in a traditional exercise program.

Tips for Maintaining Regular Physical Activity

The drop out rate for exercise programs is about 50 percent. What can you do to increase a person's likelihood of continuing to be physically active?

Reduce Boredom: Here are a few ideas to alleviate the boredom that sometimes accompanies doing the same physical activity over a long period of time:

- Try a new route. Walkers and bicyclists may want to explore another part of the neighborhood or a nearby park.

- Make physical activity part of a larger project. For example, walk to the store or work, or hop off the bus a few stops early and walk the rest of the way to your destination. Physical activity will become a healthier means of transportation.

- Use headphones. Many people enjoy listening to their favorite music or an audio book while they exercise. Headphones should not be worn if near bicycle or car traffic, nor in areas where personal safety could be jeopardized.

- Find a physical activity "buddy." Perhaps a spouse or neighbor would like some regular physical activity. Social support improves maintenance of regular physical activity habits.

- Try a new activity. It may be time to switch as a way to ward off boredom.

Regular Contact: Walking clubs offer participants regular contact with other members of the group, which can become the social support needed to continue. A telephone call to members who do not show up for a walk is an easy way to remind them to join you for the next walk.

Incentives: Incentives or prizes are frequently used to encourage people to continue physical activity programs. These can be purchased by charging small participation fees or soliciting donations from businesses in the community. Prizes can be awarded for best attendance or most improved habits. If you are recording distances or time walked, prizes also can be awarded when participants reach certain distances, e.g., 20 miles, 50 miles, etc. Incentive prizes might include t-shirts, sport watches, walking shoes, gift certificates and coupons to sporting goods stores, gym bags, sweat shirts, etc.

Overcoming Barriers to Physical Activity

There are a number of barriers to regular physical activity. Consider how you might overcome these barriers to make the program available to everyone.

Lack of Time: For your program to appeal to this group, ask program participants when is the best time for them to be physically active.

Cost: Keeping costs low is key to ensuring widespread participation. While a small membership fee may cover the cost of incentives, it may also have to be waived for some. Local businesses are often willing to donate incentives, such as t-shirts or gift certificates.

Transportation: Convenient transportation is an important issue. Is there ample parking near the walking course? Is there a bus stop nearby with frequent buses? Can participants car pool to the destination?

Safety: Not all neighborhoods are safe for activities such as walking. Community groups deal with this problem in various ways. Walking in groups and during daylight hours are good ways to enhance safety. Usually shopping malls have good security. It may be possible to work with local parks and recreation departments and the police to ensure safety in a local park. Some schools offer indoor walking opportunities.

Risks of Physical Activity: Physical activity creates some risk. Sprains, strains and other musculoskeletal injuries are common risks for the physically active. These risks can be reduced with low impact activities such as walking, biking or swimming. While sudden cardiac events can result from strenuous physical activity, this is very rare. Most health experts believe that, overall, the potential benefits of regular physical activity outweigh the risks. One method of addressing risk is through a waiver. (See sample program Waiver on page 39.)

Program Ideas

- Hold a poker walk as a kick-off for a walking campaign. Walkers receive a card at various sites along a walking route. Best hands are awarded prizes donated by merchants.

- Renovate old bikes and leave them around town or near a bike trail.

- Form a "winter wellness pack" and meet regularly during the winter/spring months (January through May) to strengthen the resolve of everyone involved. Provide shirts and log books and encourage participants to "travel" in packs.

- Work with the local city government to provide bike trails, an invaluable resource for walking, biking, etc.

- Start a local mall walkers group. These indoor areas can provide valuable fitness facilities.

- Post this sign by stairs: "Don't think of them as stairs, but as very expensive workout equipment."

- Encourage 5-times-a-week walkers by including their names in drawings for t-shirts and other prizes.

Walking programs can be creative and fun, and help establish strong social support for healthier lifestyles.

FITNESS INITIATIVES

Develop a fitness message and saturate the community with it.

- Place a "Bee Fit" message in community church bulletins and repeat for several weeks. In the spirit of a sewing bee or quilting bee, the "Bee Fit" message could suggest times to walk together.

- Approach the local paper and shopper and offer to write regular physical activity and nutrition articles. Include lists of events.

- Place bookmarks with a positive **5 Plus 5** message at libraries and book stores.

Relate the message to the calendar.

- Create book displays featuring appropriate activities during special months: bike safety during American Bike Month (May), heart-healthy habits in National Heart Month (February), and the Food Guide Pyramid in National Nutrition Month (March).

- Implement a New Year's Eve walk with healthy food and drink to support resolutions at the new year. Provide suggestions for positive, sustainable resolutions.

- Sponsor a Super Bowl party that features a pre-game walk and healthy snacks of fruit, thereby including both the "Physical Five" and the "Food Five."

- Form a group to work off extra calories during the high gain (hibernation) period from November through January.

Encourage small steps and enjoyable activities.

- Sponsor team competitions such as weight loss efforts. Award prizes for highest percentage of pounds lost by a team rather than for number of pounds lost by individuals. This places emphasis on smaller more attainable goals.

- Create certificates. With ready access to computers and print shops, it is easy and inexpensive to recognize efforts with certificates that can be either humorous ("Tired Foot" Award) or serious.

- Plan a scavenger hunt walk or bike ride. Contestants can take pictures with Polaroid cameras to show the items they have found.

• Form a walking club; it can be the key to effective change. Across the nation, walking clubs are an increasingly popular way to get in shape. Many people find the social aspect of clubs very important.

Listed on page 46 are several good sources of walking club materials. Also included as a part of this program are safety tips, activity logs and a screening questionnaire for high risk participants. These can be easily and inexpensively photocopied or printed.

How to Develop a Home-Based Exercise Program

Surveys show that many people are not willing or able to attend physical activity classes or join groups. They may still be interested in regular physical activity. Researchers at Stanford University developed a method to encourage sedentary adults to exercise using a "home-based program." They reasoned that for people who couldn't attend classes, a personalized physical activity program and regular follow-up could be an effective means to increase physical activity among sedentary adults.

The program consisted of an initial 30-minute appointment with a phone counselor to develop a personalized program and a contract that specified program details. Participants completed monthly logs recording their physical activity goals and actual performance. These logs were returned by mail to the program. Program staff telephoned participants regularly to encourage continued physical activity and to help overcome barriers.

Researchers found that after one year, about 75% of home-based participants maintained their program, while only 52% of class participants remained physically active.

The components of a home-based physical activity program include:

1. recruitment,

2. preparation,

3. appointment and

4. follow-up phone calls.

Recruitment: Advertisements in the newspaper and telephone calls are effective ways to recruit participants to a program. Post flyers at grocery stores, laundromats, community centers, or anywhere the target audience is likely to see them. Mailings or personal invitations may also be used.

Preparation: Some advance planning is required before meeting with program participants. Here is a checklist of these activities.

• Create a list of existing physical activity classes offered by organizations such as the local parks and recreation department, the YMCA/YWCA/JCC and private fitness clubs.

• Review and make copies of the forms *Physical Activity Readiness Questionnaire, Physical Activity Contract* and *Waiver.* These forms, found at the end of this section, can be personalized with your organizational logo. A few of the forms require information to be filled in before photocopying.

• Prepare handouts: Several informational handouts are included at the end of this section. They can be photocopied as they are or personalized by adding the organization's logo with a quick cut and paste job.

The Appointment: Begin with a short talk about the health benefits of the **5 Plus 5** program. There are several handouts to assist you. Stress that light to moderate physical activity can result in health benefits. A walking program, for example, is enough activity to improve health. In addition, emphasize the importance of lifelong activity. As with all habits, it is normal to stop sometimes and to begin again. Participants should not feel discouraged or guilty if they stop exercising for a time.

Complete the *Physical Activity Readiness Questionnaire (PARQ)* (see page 37). If a participant needs to see a doctor before beginning the program, arrange for another meeting to finish the intake appointment. Encourage or even assist in making the appointment with a physician.

Help participants who are completely sedentary determine their preferences for type of activity and location, and availability of equipment and other resources.

Complete the *Physical Activity Contract* (see page 38). Be specific, starting with the type of activity and location. Include days and times for proposed physical activity. The minimum goal is three times per week for 30 minutes. The ideal goal is five or six times per week for 30 minutes. Although many participants will start at a lower physical activity level, encourage them to work toward these goals.

Use a log sheet to record physical activity (see page 47). Show participants how to log progress. Ask them to complete the record sheet on a weekly basis and mail it to you at the end of the month. Provide return envelopes and postage if possible.

At the end of the appointment review safety tips, collect the signed waiver and answer any questions.

Follow-Up Telephone Calls: It is normal for people to cut back on or stop exercising. The program coordinator's role is to help the participant solve problems that interfere with physical activity. Instead of lecturing or making someone feel guilty, try to define the barriers to physical activity as clearly as possible. Brainstorm about ways to overcome the obstacles.

Consider short follow-up phone calls. The purpose of the call is to provide feedback and reinforcement for maintaining the personalized physical activity program. It may be helpful to contact participants weekly during the first month, biweekly during the second month and monthly thereafter.

Benefits of the Physical Five and Food Five

Regular activity and proper nutrition can help you
- sleep better
- maintain weight
- have more energy
- increase your sense of well being
- decrease stress

Regular activity can prevent or delay
- heart disease
- high blood pressure
- diabetes
- osteoporosis (brittle bones)

**There's more good news about physical fitness.
Even light to moderate activity can improve your health.**

Research on Physical Activity and Health

The General Benefits of Physical Activity

- Longer life spans for those who are more physically active

- Enhanced strength, flexibility, endurance and weight control

- Increased sense of well being, a greater satisfaction with body shape and weight

- Easier to prevent weight-loss regain cycles and to reverse the metabolic reduction due to chronic dieting cycles

Examples of Moderate Amounts of Activity

Washing and waxing a car for 45-60 minutes

Washing windows or floors for 45-60 minutes

Playing volleyball for 45 minutes

Gardening for 30-45 minutes

Wheeling self in wheelchair for 30-40 minutes

Walking 1 3/4 miles in 35 minutes (20 min/mile)

Basketball (shooting baskets) for 30 minutes

Bicycling 5 miles in 30 minutes

Dancing fast (social) for 30 minutes

Pushing a stroller 1 1/2 miles in 30 minutes

Raking leaves for 30 minutes

Walking 2 miles in 30 minutes (15 min/mile)

Water aerobics for 30 minutes

Swimming laps for 20 minutes

Wheelchair basketball for 20 minutes

Basketball (playing a game) for 15-20 minutes

Bicycling 4 miles in 15 minutes

Jumping rope for 15 minutes

Running 1 1/2 miles in 15 minutes (10 min/mile)

Shoveling snow for 15 minutes

Stair walking for 15 minutes

A moderate amount of physical activity is roughly equivalent to physical activity that uses approximately 150 calories of energy per day, or 1,000 calories per week.

Getting Started

Warming Up and Cooling Down

Warming up and cooling down are good ways to prevent injuries and sore muscles. This means starting slowly for the first 5-10 minutes of your workout and then increasing your pace. Save 5-10 minutes at the end of your workout to go slowly again, or to cool down.

Shoes and Equipment

Avoid injuries by wearing the right shoes and using the right equipment. For most people, a good pair of walking or running shoes is the only equipment necessary. Get shoes with good heels, arch supports, and plenty of room to wiggle your toes. Before you buy new athletic shoes, make sure they fit comfortably. If you are using other equipment, such as a stationary bicycle, make sure it is well maintained and in good working order.

Getting Started

Which type of activity is best?

Almost any aerobic activity will get you into shape because it means moving your large muscle groups rhythmically. This requires you to breathe more rapidly and increases your heart rate. Walking, swimming, bicycling, climbing stairs and rowing are just some of the aerobic activities that can improve your cardiovascular health.

Finding the right pace.

Moderate physical activity can improve health. This means you don't have to maintain the fastest pace possible in order to get healthier. One way to set the right pace is to imagine a scale from one to ten. One is the equivalent of sitting on the couch and ten is moving as fast as you possibly can. A moderate pace is right in between. When you are *starting* a fitness program, aim for a five on the scale.

1	2	3	4	5	6	7	8	9	10
Couch potato				Just right					Fastest pace

Try the "talk test." If you can't talk while doing your specific physical activity, it's a sign that you are working too hard. Slow down.

Research on Physical Activity and Heart Health

- Those who are sedentary are about two times as likely to develop coronary heart disease (CHD) as those who are active. Those who are sedentary have a 50% higher chance of dying from CHD than those who are active.

- People who are less physically active have almost twice the risk of developing hypertension as those who are active.

- An active childhood, without continued activity in adulthood, will not protect adults from CHD. Athletes who were studied maintained low rates of CHD only if they remained active later in life.

Research on Physical Activity and Health

Activity and the Prevention of Other Health Problems

• Physical activity can help in the prevention and treatment of several common chronic health problems: non-insulin dependent diabetes mellitus, hypertension, obesity, peripheral vascular disease and depression.

• There is some evidence to suggest that being sedentary may increase the risk of developing some types of cancer, particularly cancer of the colon and the female reproductive system.

• Physical activity strengthens bones, increases bone density and may reduce the risk of fractures in the elderly.

Physical Activity Readiness Questionnaire

Light to moderate physical activity is safe for most people. This questionnaire will help determine whether you can begin your program immediately or whether you should consult your doctor first.

Do you have any of these conditions?

- Heart trouble, heart murmur or coronary heart disease;

- Pains or pressure in your left or mid-chest area, left neck, shoulder or arm during or right after exertion;

- Frequent faint or dizzy spells;

- Diabetes;

- Uncontrolled high blood pressure (over 140/90);

- Arthritis or other problems with bones and joints;

- Are you over 50 and not used to exercising?

CAUTION:
If any of the above apply to you, talk to your doctor before beginning your new program.

Physical Activity Contract

I am ready to begin my new program.

I will _____ _____ each week for _____ minutes each day.
           (activity)   (times)   (number)

I will be at/in _____.
                                   (location)

The best days for me are   M T W TH F S SN   from _____.
                            (days)   (times)

If I have any questions or problems, I know that I can telephone my counselor,

_____ at _____.
             (name)   (telephone number)

I understand that my counselor will call me on _____ at _____
                                          (date)   (time)

to discuss my new program.

_____ _____
            (signature)   (date)

Waiver

This project is under the direction of

_____ .

I understand that the benefits from participating in this group include learning more about the benefits of an active lifestyle and meeting my own goals.

I state that I am free from heart disease and other medical conditions, or that I have written permission from my doctor to participate in this program.

I release the sponsoring organization(s) and personnel from any responsibility or liability for any injury or health consequences that may result from my participation in this program.

My signature indicates that I have full knowledge of the purpose of the program, the benefits I may expect and the risks involved. I agree to participate on this basis.

_____   _____
(signature)   (date)

_____   _____
(address)   (telephone #)

Safety Tips

The Weather

On hot days, slow down your routine until you get used to the heat. When the temperature is 90 degrees or above, exercise during the early morning hours or in the evening. Drink lots of water. The signs of heat stroke include dizziness, weakness and becoming very tired. Sweating often stops and one's body temperature can become dangerously high.

On cold days, wear several layers of clothing. Take off layers as you warm up. Wearing a hat is important as well. Up to 40 percent of body heat loss occurs through your head and neck.

When to Stop

The "talk test" is a good way to tell if your pace is too fast. If you can do your routine and talk, your pace is about right. If you are too out of breath to talk, slow down.

Contact your physician immediately if you feel suddenly dizzy, faint or break into a cold sweat, or if you feel pain or pressure in your left or mid-chest area, left neck, shoulder or arm.

General Safety

If you are outside, walk or run against traffic. Bike with traffic. In the evening, find a safe, well-lit place to go. Being with others is a good strategy to improve your safety at night. Wear good supportive shoes and clothes that "breathe."

THE FOOD FIVE: NUTRITION PROGRAM STRATEGIES

Imagine starting a health promotion program that can make a difference in your community. With its simple message and clearly defined goals, the **5 A Day** for Better Health Program has become the "Food Five" in the **5 Plus 5** physical activity/nutrition program.

Background Information

The national **5 A Day** Program has a simple, positive message: *eat at least five servings of fruits and vegetables each day as part of a high-fiber, low-fat diet.*

The national **5 A Day** Program is distinctive as a partnership between government and the food industry. It is sponsored jointly by the National Cancer Institute (NCI), a government agency of the U.S. Department of Health and Human Services, and the Produce for Better Health Foundation (PBH), an independent, nonprofit consumer education foundation of the fruit and vegetable industry.

Program Ideas

Ideas and efforts to combine the "Food Five" and the "Physical Five" will make a tremendous impact on the community. The following pages contain lists of suggested places to conduct the Food Five activities, ways to communicate about **5 Plus 5** events and specific suggestions for community **5 Plus 5** programs. Involve community partners in planning, implementing and evaluating all **5 Plus 5** program activities. Use imagination and have fun spreading this important message!

Places For 5 Plus 5 Activities

Listed below are some places where the 5 Plus 5 message could be communicated. Select those that work best for you!

State/Local Events
carnivals
commodity festivals
concerts
health fairs
shopping malls
state agriculture fairs

Food Distribution
cafeterias
farmer's markets
grocery stores
hospitals
long-term care facilities
Meals on Wheels
schools
senior centers
company cafeterias

Sporting Events
baseball games
softball games
basketball games
football games
fitness centers
Little League
softball leagues
swimming pools
soccer games

Civic Community Services
Boy Scouts/Girl Scouts
Jaycees
Rotary Clubs
museums
town parades
community festivals
YMCA/YWCA/JCC
4-H/FFA
other service groups (Lions, Elks, etc.)

Businesses
bulletin boards
checkout counters
coffee break rooms
dentists' offices
doctors' offices
lunch rooms
waiting rooms

Religious Events
church socials
church newsletters
church programs
fund-raisers
activity groups

Diet Centers
health clubs
Weight Watchers

Media
advertisements
books
disc jockeys
food writers
health writers
magazines
newspapers
other media
news editors
sports figures
weather people

Local Health Groups
American Cancer Society
American Diabetes Association
American Heart Association
Public Health Office
County Extension Service

5 Plus 5 Communications Tools

Listed below are various tools that can be used to communicate the **5 Plus 5** message in many of the places listed on the previous page. Some tools will simply inform people of the need to eat 5 daily servings of fruits and vegetables. Others will actually motivate behavior change. **Use the method that will work best for your audience.**

To create awareness, try...
ad copy
ads
answering machine messages
badges
balloons
billboards
books
brochures
bulletin boards
bumper stickers
buttons
displays
electronic mail
exhibits
faxes
fund-raisers
hats
magazines
mascots
newsletters
newspapers
posters
press releases
PSAs
radio
receipt stubs
slide presentations
songs
sweatshirts
t-shirts
television
video

To motivate consumers, try...
awards
contests
rewards
school field trips
taste-testings

To develop skills, try...
cooking demonstrations
food handling demos
how to select low-fat fruit and
    vegetable menu items
how to select low-fat fruit and
    vegetable snacks
recipes
tours

To provide social support, try...
developing a buddy system
encouraging family/friends
giving fruit and vegetable gift baskets

To provide environmental support, try...
convenient fruits and vegetables
offering meals and menus with more
    fruits and vegetables
ready-to-eat fruits and vegetables
offering snacks with more fruits
    and vegetables
local and state proclamations
vending machines

Ideas For Activities

Grocers may have limited time to devote to projects, but often become enthusiastic partners. Perhaps they will donate products or money for a project, or put you in touch with suppliers who will. Since grocery stores are (or can be) participants in the **5 A Day** Program, they may be able to donate **5 A Day** promotional materials or brochures for **5 Plus 5** activities.

Awareness Activities

Encourage your grocer to use creative displays: Place **5 A Day** signs in the fruit and vegetable section of the frozen food aisle; set up end-aisle or checkout displays with ice buckets containing bags of precut carrots or juice; place **5 A Day** and **5 Plus 5** brochures at the front door, at the checkout, and next to in-store circulars.

Product donations: Help your grocer hold a canned fruit and vegetable drive for a charitable group or Food Bank as part of a **5 Plus 5** event. Many community groups (Jaycees, scouts, etc.) are excellent at setting up events and may be willing to help. Encourage local grocers to donate products and **5 A Day** brochures to help create awareness. Point out that the added publicity will help draw attention to the grocery store with minimal effort on the grocer's part.

Conduct in-store polls: Allow consumers to "vote" for their favorite fruits and vegetables. Take polls throughout the store to include fresh, frozen, dried and canned produce. Promote a daily tabulation to health reporters and the media. Give a "cents-off" coupon to voters.

Radio coverage: Involve local radio stations. Work with them and your grocer to set up a live remote from the grocery store or other activity location. The grocer can advertise sale items while they announce your event.

Print publicity: Help your grocery store's public relations or consumer affairs professional develop a press release to send to local media about joint **5 Plus 5** activities.

Community attention: Ask to block off a section of the grocery store parking lot as the end or beginning of a **5 Plus 5** fun run to generate excitement and pull in passing traffic.

Television coverage: Notify local radio and television stations in your area about **5 A Day Week** events and other **5 Plus 5** promotions. Ask your grocer or local growers to donate fruit and vegetable baskets to give to local television personalities; bring your mayor into the store to officially proclaim **5 A Day Week** in your town or kick off a **5 Plus 5** event.

Motivation Activities

Promote convenience: Conduct food demonstrations of quick **5 A Day** recipes.

Raffles and contests: Help your grocer arrange to hold a raffle in the produce department every 5 hours for a week; give every 55th customer $5 off their fruit and vegetable purchase; offer every 555th customer a $55 fruit and vegetable shopping spree – fresh, frozen, canned or dried. Check with authorities regarding the legality of and/or licensing requirements for holding raffles or contests.

Make it memorable: Have the grocery store promote a farmer's market theme in the parking lot with tents, flowers, fruits and vegetables, hay bales, etc.; place picnic tables and juice bars outside the store. Promote **5 Plus 5** at local farmer's markets.

Incentives: Encourage local grocers to offer coupons or sales on fruits and vegetables for customers. Try conducting 5 for $1 sales, or buy 5 – get one free. Help promote the activities.

Promote the program: Assist retailers with food demonstrations. Use sampling, demonstrations, or tip cards to remind consumers that the **5 A Day** goal is not a difficult one. Show how fruits and vegetables can be combined with non-fat dips or seasonings, added to entrees, or included in healthy soups or other easy meals.

Walking Resources:

American Association of Retired Persons (AARP)
601 E. Street NW
Washington, DC 20049
(202) 434-2230 or (202) 434-AARP

Provides a free walking club and event organizational guide, *Step by Step: Planning Walking Activities.* Addresses recruitment, safety and dealing with obstacles.

The American Volkssport Association
1001 Pat Booker Road, Suite 101
Universal City, TX 78148
(210) 659-2112

Various materials related to, and promoting, walking.

National Organization of Mall Walkers
P.O. Box 256
Hermann, MO 65041
Phone & Fax: (573) 486-3945

Walking Magazine
9-11 Harcourt Street
Boston, MA 02116
Attn: Walking Tip Sheet

Send a self-addressed, stamped envelope to receive a copy of *Walking Tip Sheet.*

Nutrition Resources:

Centers for Disease Control and Prevention
National Center for Chronic Disease Prevention and Health Promotion
Division of Nutrition and Physical Activity, MS K-46
4770 Buford Highway, NE
Atlanta, GA 30341
(888) CDC-4NRG or (888) 232-4674
http://www.cdc.gov

Provides extensive information on coalition building, nutrition and physical activity.

Produce for Better Health Foundation
5301 Limestone Road, Suite 101
Wilmington, DE 19808
(302) 235-2329
Fax: (302) 235-5555

Apparel, posters, brochures and official **5 A Day** Program recipes are available from this nonprofit foundation of the produce industry. As the industry partner in the **5 A Day** Program, PBH sublicenses grocery stores, food suppliers and merchandisers, restaurants and other food service businesses in the program, and they sell program starter kits and other program materials.

Remline Corporation
139 East Chestnut Hill Road
Newark, DE 19713
(800) 555-6115

Remline is the official supplier of **5 A Day** apparel (t-shirts, sweatshirts, aprons, hats, etc.), buttons, refrigerator magnets, key chains and other premium and promotional items.

Try-Foods International, Inc.
207 Semoran Commerce Place
P.O. Drawer 2248
Apopka, FL 32704-2248
(800) 421-8871

Try-Foods supplies official **5 A Day** brochures, stickers, posters, videos and other promotional materials.

TIP: When reproducing for handouts, copy pages 47 and 48 back to back.

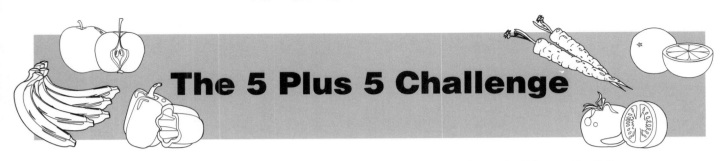

The 5 Plus 5 Challenge

Physical Activity

Enjoy 30 minutes of physical activity at least five days each week. Each square represents 10 continuous minutes of physical activity. Check off one square each time you engage in 10 minutes of physical activity.

Fruits & Vegetables

Eat five or more servings of fruits and vegetables each day. Check off a square each time you eat a serving of fruits or vegetables.

	Physical Activity	Fruits & Vegetables
Monday	☐ ☐ ☐	☐ ☐ ☐ ☐ ☐
Tuesday	☐ ☐ ☐	☐ ☐ ☐ ☐ ☐
Wednesday	☐ ☐ ☐	☐ ☐ ☐ ☐ ☐
Thursday	☐ ☐ ☐	☐ ☐ ☐ ☐ ☐
Friday	☐ ☐ ☐	☐ ☐ ☐ ☐ ☐
Saturday	☐ ☐ ☐	☐ ☐ ☐ ☐ ☐
Sunday	☐ ☐ ☐	☐ ☐ ☐ ☐ ☐
Monday	☐ ☐ ☐	☐ ☐ ☐ ☐ ☐
Tuesday	☐ ☐ ☐	☐ ☐ ☐ ☐ ☐
Wednesday	☐ ☐ ☐	☐ ☐ ☐ ☐ ☐
Thursday	☐ ☐ ☐	☐ ☐ ☐ ☐ ☐
Friday	☐ ☐ ☐	☐ ☐ ☐ ☐ ☐
Saturday	☐ ☐ ☐	☐ ☐ ☐ ☐ ☐
Sunday	☐ ☐ ☐	☐ ☐ ☐ ☐ ☐
Monday	☐ ☐ ☐	☐ ☐ ☐ ☐ ☐
Tuesday	☐ ☐ ☐	☐ ☐ ☐ ☐ ☐
Wednesday	☐ ☐ ☐	☐ ☐ ☐ ☐ ☐

	Physical Activity	Fruits & Vegetables
Thursday	☐ ☐ ☐	☐ ☐ ☐ ☐ ☐
Friday	☐ ☐ ☐	☐ ☐ ☐ ☐ ☐
Saturday	☐ ☐ ☐	☐ ☐ ☐ ☐ ☐
Sunday	☐ ☐ ☐	☐ ☐ ☐ ☐ ☐
Monday	☐ ☐ ☐	☐ ☐ ☐ ☐ ☐
Tuesday	☐ ☐ ☐	☐ ☐ ☐ ☐ ☐
Wednesday	☐ ☐ ☐	☐ ☐ ☐ ☐ ☐
Thursday	☐ ☐ ☐	☐ ☐ ☐ ☐ ☐
Friday	☐ ☐ ☐	☐ ☐ ☐ ☐ ☐
Saturday	☐ ☐ ☐	☐ ☐ ☐ ☐ ☐
Sunday	☐ ☐ ☐	☐ ☐ ☐ ☐ ☐
Monday	☐ ☐ ☐	☐ ☐ ☐ ☐ ☐
Tuesday	☐ ☐ ☐	☐ ☐ ☐ ☐ ☐
Wednesday	☐ ☐ ☐	☐ ☐ ☐ ☐ ☐
Thursday	☐ ☐ ☐	☐ ☐ ☐ ☐ ☐
Friday	☐ ☐ ☐	☐ ☐ ☐ ☐ ☐
Saturday	☐ ☐ ☐	☐ ☐ ☐ ☐ ☐

Participant Name _____ **Return to** _____

SAMPLE HANDOUT

TIP: When reproducing for handouts, copy pages 47 and 48 back to back.

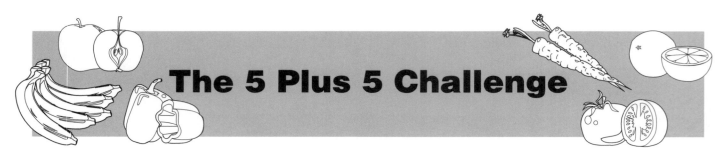

The 5 Plus 5 Challenge

Physical Activity

Enjoy 30 minutes of physical activity at least five days each week. Each square represents 10 continuous minutes of physical activity. Check off one square each time you engage in 10 minutes of physical activity.

Fruits & Vegetables

Eat five or more servings of fruits and vegetables each day. Check off a square each time you eat a serving of fruits or vegetables.

	Physical Activity	Fruits & Vegetables
Sunday	☐ ☐ ☐	☐ ☐ ☐ ☐ ☐
Monday	☐ ☐ ☐	☐ ☐ ☐ ☐ ☐
Tuesday	☐ ☐ ☐	☐ ☐ ☐ ☐ ☐
Wednesday	☐ ☐ ☐	☐ ☐ ☐ ☐ ☐
Thursday	☐ ☐ ☐	☐ ☐ ☐ ☐ ☐
Friday	☐ ☐ ☐	☐ ☐ ☐ ☐ ☐
Saturday	☐ ☐ ☐	☐ ☐ ☐ ☐ ☐
Sunday	☐ ☐ ☐	☐ ☐ ☐ ☐ ☐
Monday	☐ ☐ ☐	☐ ☐ ☐ ☐ ☐
Tuesday	☐ ☐ ☐	☐ ☐ ☐ ☐ ☐
Wednesday	☐ ☐ ☐	☐ ☐ ☐ ☐ ☐
Thursday	☐ ☐ ☐	☐ ☐ ☐ ☐ ☐
Friday	☐ ☐ ☐	☐ ☐ ☐ ☐ ☐
Saturday	☐ ☐ ☐	☐ ☐ ☐ ☐ ☐
Sunday	☐ ☐ ☐	☐ ☐ ☐ ☐ ☐
Monday	☐ ☐ ☐	☐ ☐ ☐ ☐ ☐
Tuesday	☐ ☐ ☐	☐ ☐ ☐ ☐ ☐

	Physical Activity	Fruits & Vegetables
Wednesday	☐ ☐ ☐	☐ ☐ ☐ ☐ ☐
Thursday	☐ ☐ ☐	☐ ☐ ☐ ☐ ☐
Friday	☐ ☐ ☐	☐ ☐ ☐ ☐ ☐
Saturday	☐ ☐ ☐	☐ ☐ ☐ ☐ ☐
Sunday	☐ ☐ ☐	☐ ☐ ☐ ☐ ☐
Monday	☐ ☐ ☐	☐ ☐ ☐ ☐ ☐
Tuesday	☐ ☐ ☐	☐ ☐ ☐ ☐ ☐
Wednesday	☐ ☐ ☐	☐ ☐ ☐ ☐ ☐
Thursday	☐ ☐ ☐	☐ ☐ ☐ ☐ ☐
Friday	☐ ☐ ☐	☐ ☐ ☐ ☐ ☐
Saturday	☐ ☐ ☐	☐ ☐ ☐ ☐ ☐
Sunday	☐ ☐ ☐	☐ ☐ ☐ ☐ ☐
Monday	☐ ☐ ☐	☐ ☐ ☐ ☐ ☐
Tuesday	☐ ☐ ☐	☐ ☐ ☐ ☐ ☐
Wednesday	☐ ☐ ☐	☐ ☐ ☐ ☐ ☐
Thursday	☐ ☐ ☐	☐ ☐ ☐ ☐ ☐
Friday	☐ ☐ ☐	☐ ☐ ☐ ☐ ☐

Participant Name _____ **Return to** _____

TIP: When reproducing for handouts, copy pages 49 and 50 back to back.

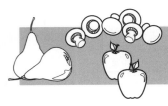
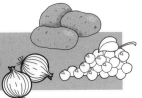

The 5 Plus 5 Challenge

Participant Registration

PARTICIPANT	ADDRESS	PHONE NUMBER
1.		
2.		
3.		
4.		
5.		
6.		
7.		
8.		
9.		
10.		
11.		
12.		
13.		
14.		
15.		
16.		
17.		
18.		
19.		
20.		
21.		
22.		
23.		
24.		
25.		
26.		

PARTICIPANT	ADDRESS	PHONE NUMBER
27.		
28.		
29.		
30.		
31.		
32.		
33.		
34.		
35.		
36.		
37.		
38.		
39.		
40.		
41.		
42.		
43.		
44.		
45.		
46.		
47.		
48.		
49.		
50.		
51.		
52.		
53.		
54.		
55.		
56.		

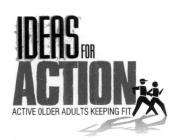

IDEAS FOR ACTION
ACTIVE OLDER ADULTS KEEPING FIT

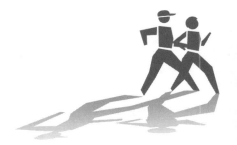

Line Dancing For Seniors

Organization: Leroy Springs Recreation Complex
P.O. Box 280
Ft. Mills, SC 29716
Phone: (803) 547-1045
Fax: (803) 547-3273
Contributor: Donna Wilson, Senior Citizens Director
(Jan Martin, Current Senior Citizens Director)

Program Objective

• to promote an active, fun, no-cost program for Seniors

Materials/Equipment Needed

• appropriate music
• tape player
• room large enough to dance in (aerobics or dance studio with mirrors ideal, but not necessary)

Procedures and Teaching Strategies

• lots of repetition – don't move too fast

Repeat the same dances a lot and add new dances slowly. Give written instructions. You may want to change the music or alter the steps of popular line dances to make them more appropriate (slower, easier) for Seniors. Encourage participants to stick with it and not to get discouraged. Don't be too serious. Praise participants, but also tease them when they make mistakes – laugh a lot! After class, help them individually with steps they had difficulty learning. Class participants also help each other, especially the new students.

Program Description

This is a 45-minute weekly ongoing class offered to Seniors in line dancing. This class is basically the same as any line dance class, but because it is geared toward Senior participants, they feel very comfortable around their peers, and appreciate the fact that this class is specifically for them.

Program Results

This class was started two years ago. The number of participants has tripled, and the more they dance, the better they are at it. Class participants even learn new dances more quickly.

This has been a very successful program. We were able to offer this class at no expense to participants, and at very little expense to the center.

Program Tips

- **Tie in class time with social events.** For example, this class is held each week on the same morning the Senior Citizen's Club meets for a luncheon.

- **Perform** at area nursing homes, county and state fairs, malls, parades, etc.

- **Dance space should be carpet free**, if possible. Carpet can impede lateral movement and cause footing problems.

- If a carpeted area is used, **avoid patterned carpet**, as it can cause visual/balance problems.

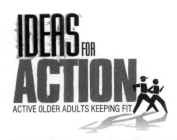

IDEAS FOR ACTION
ACTIVE OLDER ADULTS KEEPING FIT

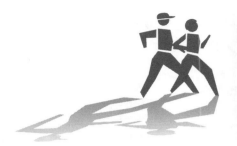

Maple Knoll Wellness Center

Organization: Maple Knoll Village
11100 Springfield Pike
Cincinnati, OH 45246
Phone: (513) 782-4340
Fax: (513) 782-4324
Contributor: Jan Montague, M.G.S., Director

Program Objectives

• to take a total approach to wellness

• to teach that wellness is more than fitness; it is an attitude, a way of life

Materials/Equipment Needed

Maple Knoll Wellness Center is approximately 8,500 square feet and includes:

• warm water swimming pool

• whirlpool

• group activity room

• meditation areas

• men's and women's locker rooms

• exercise room equipment includes Keiser strength-training equipment, Nu-Step recumbent steppers, Cybex multi-column unit and treadmills, exercise bench, hand weights and dynabands

Procedures and Teaching Strategies

The Six Dimensions of Wellness

Maple Knoll Wellness Center instructors have been trained to guide members through the process of examining each facet of life. Together, staff and members determine which dimension needs development or improvement. Then, individualized action plans, time lines and goals are established. Since wellness is progressive and ongoing, the program is not static. Areas within the center are staffed by trained professionals.

Emotional: Emphasizes an awareness and acceptance of one's feelings. It reflects the degree to which an individual feels positive and enthusiastic about one's self and life.

- Control stress
- Express emotions
- Accept feelings
- Manage success
- Manage failure

Physical: Promotes participation in activities for cardiovascular endurance, muscular strengthening and flexibility.

- Fitness
- Nutrition
- Prevention/health screenings
- Daily activities
- Lifestyle habits

Intellectual: Promotes the use of one's mind to create a greater understanding and appreciation of oneself and others.

- Lifetime learning
- New challenges
- Creativity
- Exploration

Social: Emphasizes the creation and maintenance of healthy relationships.

- Interaction with others
- Interaction with environment
- Respect for others
- Tolerance of differences

Spiritual: Involves seeking meaning and purpose in human existence.

- Morals
- Values
- Ethics
- Meaning
- Purpose

Vocational: Emphasizes the process of determining and achieving personal and occupational interests.

- Occupation
- Abilities
- Goals
- Interests
- Personal mission

All areas of the wellness center are staffed by trained and certified professionals. In addition to holding bachelor's and master's degrees in disciplines such as exercise science and gerontology, the staff is certified in fitness programming, CPR and water safety.

Maple Knoll Wellness Center also conducts professional training programs for the American Senior Fitness Association, Arthritis Aquatic Certification and the Aquatic Exercise Association.

HOURS OF OPERATION

Maple Knoll Village Residents and Center for Older Adult Members may use the facility during the following time periods:

M W F	6:30 am -	7:00 pm
T Th	9:00 am -	7:00 pm
Sa	8:30 am -	12:30 pm

Maple Knoll Village Employees may use the facility during the following time periods:

M W F	6:30 am -	9:30 am
	11:00 am -	2:00 pm
	3:00 pm -	7:00 pm
T Th	11:00 am -	2:00 pm
	3:00 pm -	7:00 pm
Sa	8:30 am -	12:30 pm

Program Description

Maple Knoll Wellness Center is located on the campus of Maple Knoll Village, a nationally accredited, continuing care retirement community of some 650 residents age 55 and older in the Springdale area of Cincinnati, Ohio.

Opened in 1995, the Maple Knoll Wellness Center was developed to serve those 55 and older. Research shows that taking part in a fitness program improves health and slows the aging process. To maintain optimum health, however, people need more than just physical exercise. All facets of their being – mind, spirit, and body – must be exercised to realize their maximum potential. Programs and classes provided at the Maple Knoll Wellness Center adhere to a human-wholeness principle.

Program Results

Jan Montague, Director of Maple Knoll Village Wellness Center, states, "We owe it to our membership and to the general public to demonstrate what a holistic program is all about. We are training individuals to care for themselves. Some are young at 90, while others are old at 60."

Program Tips

- **Allow a lot of space** around each piece of exercise equipment to accommodate wheelchairs and walkers.

- **Choose equipment that is versatile** in order to meet the needs of a variety of individuals.

Note: Contact Jan Montague in regard to consultation services for retirement communities. See *Senior Fitness Consultants* in the *Resource* section of this manual.

Maple Knoll
Wellness Center Model

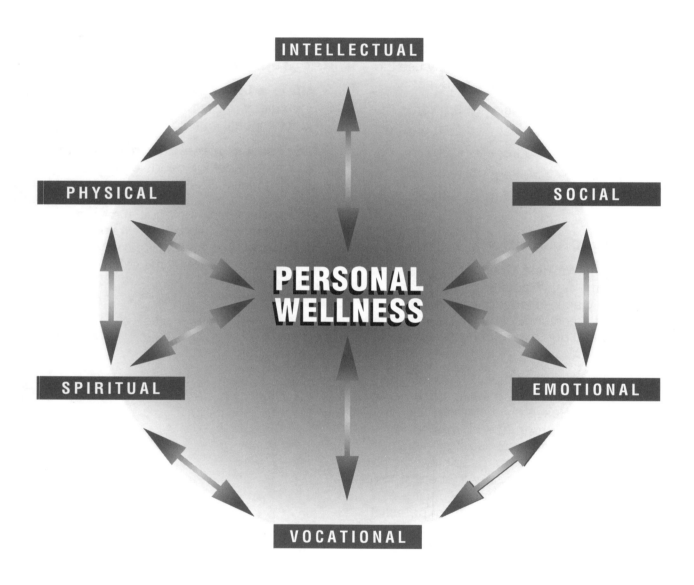

TIP: To create a brochure, copy pages 57 and 58 back to back.

Maple Knoll Wellness Center presents...

"ENERGIZE YOUR LIFE!"

An Exercise Class for the Body, Mind & Spirit

Mondays and Wednesdays 9:00 - 10:00 am

Maple Knoll Center for Older Adults

11199 Springfield Pike

Free to Wellness Center members $2.50/Non-members

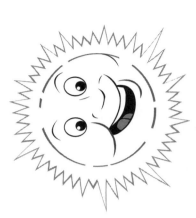

Maple Knoll Wellness Center
Where Health is More Than Fitness

In concert with the "Energize Your Life" connection of Body/Mind/Spirit, the Maple Knoll Wellness Center reflects a philosophy that emphasizes a holistic approach to health promotion. Comprehensive programming encourages participants to continually develop, improve and balance all six dimensions: emotional, intellectual, physical, spiritual, social and vocational. Aspects from each of the dimensions are integrated into all phases of programming.

Here are a few of the programs offered at the Wellness Center:

- Tai Chi
- Yoga
- Whirlpool
- Warm Water Pool (89°)
- Strength Training and Cardiovascular Equipment
- Reflexology
- Massage Therapy
- Lifetime Learning Lectures
- Out-patient Physical Therapy

If you would like further information, please call (513) 782-4340.

ENERGIZE YOUR LIFE!!

About the class... The format is unique in that it is designed with the older adult as the centerpiece. The class is challenging yet effective, fun and creative. There are exercises targeting full range of motion, balance, agility, strength, relaxation, deep breathing, flexibility and mind/body awareness. Each class ends with a "Thought for the Day," which could be anything from a story to a poem to a meditation. It is offered to provide each person with a different view on things that may otherwise be taken for granted. Or, just to make you laugh, smile and think.

About the instructor... The class is taught by Tony Poggiali, who is an exercise physiologist at the Maple Knoll Wellness Center. Tony is a firm believer in the principles he teaches – the mind, body and spirit are not three separate entities. When all three are fused together in perfect harmony and balance, a person can truly be free of limitations and, in accordance, achieve optimal health. Tony is heavily influenced by the practices of the East, especially Taoism.

TIP: To create a brochure, copy pages 57 and 58 back to back.

This isn't your typical exercise class...

- Storytelling
- Strength Training
- Deep Breathing Exercises
- Meditation
- Body Movement & Awareness
- Flexibility
- Mindfulness
- Philosophy

- Social Atmosphere
- Enlightenment
- Gentle Warm Up/Cool Down
- Fun!!

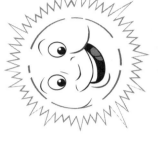

Happiness

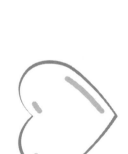

Love

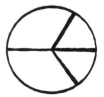

Peace

MAPLE KNOLL

Wellness Center

(Issue Number Here)   Where Health Is More Than Fitness   (513) 782-4340
September 1997

Wellness Awareness

The word *Wellness* is used by a variety of people and organizations to mean several things. To some it means health, to others it means the body, mind and spirit connection. For Maple Knoll Wellness Center members, it means the integration and balance of the six dimensions of wellness: physical, spiritual, emotional, social, intellectual and vocational. To achieve personal wellness, these dimensions must be continually developed and integrated into one's life. To begin your personal *Journey into Wellness*, listen to your inner voice. You innately know what is needed to keep yourself balanced and living at an optimal level. Unfortunately, we often tune out the messages from our inner voice. We ignore the messages because we are too busy, too tired, too overwhelmed or too stressed. Instead, be open to the needs of your body, mind and spirit; listen to the signals they are sending. For example, one day you might notice that you are more tired than usual, but you decide to press on and keep busy. Was your body trying to tell you to rest and you failed to listen? For a moment each day, pay attention to your feelings and needs. Then give yourself what your inner voice is asking to receive.

Did You Know?

Swimming Stroke Analysis

(Date)
(Time)
(Please sign up at the office.)

Come join us as we help each other learn how to swim more efficiently. This class will highlight swimming techniques to make your swimming workout more beneficial.

Did You Know?

Energize Your Life!

Mondays & Wednesdays – 9:00 - 10:00 AM
Center for Older Adults
Free to Wellness Center members – ($2.50/class non-members)

NEW CLASS!

Starting Monday, September 15, the Senior Center will be offering a program that will combine exercises for your body, mind and spirit. This one-hour class will be taught by our own Wellness Center staff member, Tony Poggiali.

Tony will lead the class through exercises emphasizing the five components of physical fitness: cardiovascular endurance, muscular strength and endurance, agility and flexibility. The course will also include programming for mental awareness and spiritual enlightenment.

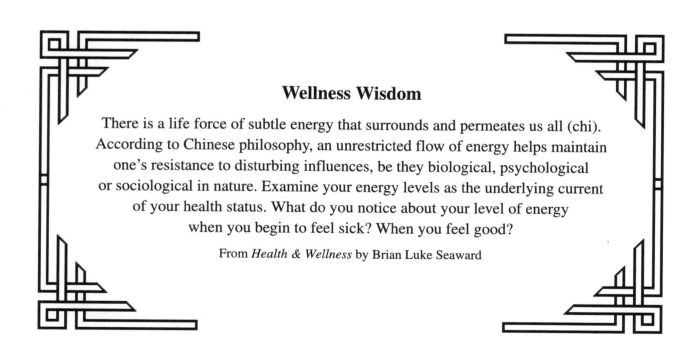

Wellness Wisdom

There is a life force of subtle energy that surrounds and permeates us all (chi). According to Chinese philosophy, an unrestricted flow of energy helps maintain one's resistance to disturbing influences, be they biological, psychological or sociological in nature. Examine your energy levels as the underlying current of your health status. What do you notice about your level of energy when you begin to feel sick? When you feel good?

From *Health & Wellness* by Brian Luke Seaward

Maple Knoll

Wellness Fair

(Date Here)
(Time Here)
Center for Older Adults
11199 Springfield Pike

At Maple Knoll, we encourage a holistic approach to health promotion. Visit the Wellness Fair to learn more about your health and wellness options.

Aromatherapy

Blood Pressure & Glucose Screening $2.00

Massage Therapy

Tai Chi

Call the Wellness Center at 782-4340 for more information.

September	"Daily" Wellness Programs	1997
	(Members Only)	

Tai Chi

Tuesday   10:30 - 11:30 AM

Wednesday   4:00 - 5:00 PM

(Assembly Room B)

Beginners YOGA

Thursdays 10:30 - 11:45 AM

(Assembly Room B)

Group Circuit Training

Tuesday and Thursday
9:30 - 10:30 AM
(Individual Exercise Room)

Walking Group

Tuesday and Thursday
11:30 - 12:30 PM
(Meet in the Wellness Center Lobby)

Flex & Tone

Tuesday and Thursday

3:15 - 4:00 PM

(Meet in the Wellness Center Lobby)

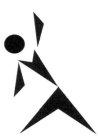

September "Daily" Wellness Programs 1997

(Members Only)

Aquatic Schedule

1 Arthritis

Monday, Wednesday, Friday
10:30 - 11:15 AM & 1:30 - 2:15 PM

Tuesday and Thursday
1:30 - 2:15 PM

2 Water Walking

Monday, Wednesday
8:45 - 9:15 AM

Tuesday and Thursday
10:30 - 11:15 AM & 2:30 - 3:15 PM

Saturday
10:30 - 11:15 AM

3 Aqua-Lite

Monday, Wednesday, Friday
2:30 - 3:15 PM

Tuesday and Thursday
9:30 - 10:15 PM

Bingo Water Exercise

Tuesday and Thursday
3:30 - 4:15 PM

(Using water noodles)

4 Aqua-Aerobics

Monday, Wednesday, Friday
9:30 - 10:15 AM

All Aquatic classes have an assigned level. Level 1 is the beginner level, and the intensity of the class increases the higher the level gets. Level 4 is our hardest class. All participants must take a level 1, 2, & 3 class before entering Level 4.

Journey into Wellness

The Wonderful World of Dreams
September 3, 10, 17, 24: *Wednesdays*
1:00 - 2:30 PM
Assembly Room B
Must Pre-Register!

Remember to SIGN UP!

Shelley Johnson, CCHt, CtHA, will present this 4-week course on dreams. Participants will learn the basics of how to use dreams to assist in their personal and spiritual growth. Cost $25.

Everything you need to know about Osteoporosis Screenings
September 3, *Wednesday*
3:00 - 4:00 PM
Assembly Room B
(Open to the Public)

John Hartman, from In-Office Bone Densitometry, will discuss the osteoporosis screening process. The Wellness Center plans to have osteoporosis screenings available at the Wellness Fair on September 16.

Laugh it Off
September 9, *Tuesday*
1:00 - 2:30 PM
Assembly Room B
(Open to the Public)

Beth Hollaender, RDLD, invites you to bring a funny joke to this meeting.
Join us as we reach our healthy weight.

Table Massage
September 12 & 26, *Fridays*
9:00 AM - 2:00 PM
Outpatient Physical Therapy Room
(Members Only)
Must Pre-Register!

Remember to SIGN UP!

Ken Kramer, LMT, will offer half-hour table massages for $20. Table massage is a great way to address all areas of the body. *Massage can be administered with clothing on.*

Journey into Wellness

Good Grief – A Bereavement Support Group
September 16, *Tuesday*
1:30 - 3:00 PM
Family Meeting Room
(Open to the Public)

Compassion and love are shared here in a warm and caring way.

Humanistic Astrology – A Personal & Practical Approach
September 22, *Monday*
1:00 - 2:00 PM
Assembly Room B
(Open to the Public)

Michael Booth will discuss how to use astrology to better understand your interpersonal relationships.

Hours of Operation

*Maple Knoll Village Residents and Center for Older Adult Members may use the facility during the following time periods:

Monday, Wednesday, Friday	6:30 AM - 7:00 PM
Tuesday and Thursday	9:00 AM - 7:00 PM
Saturday	8:30 AM - 12:30 PM

*Maple Knoll Village Employees may use the facility during the following time periods:

Monday, Wednesday, Friday	6:30 AM - 9:00 AM
	11:00 AM - 2:00 PM
	3:00 PM - 7:00 PM
Tuesday and Thursday	11:00 AM - 2:00 PM
	3:00 PM - 7:00 PM
Saturday	8:30 AM - 12:30 PM

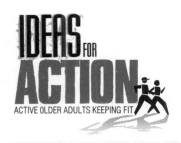

ACTIVE OLDER ADULTS KEEPING FIT

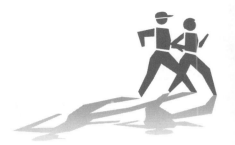

Moving Targets

Organization: SuperTarget Pharmacy Dept.
3201 Iowa Street
Lawrence, KS 66046
Phone: (785) 832-0312
Fax: (785) 832-1470
Contributor: Cyndy Herod, Registered Pharmacist

Program Objectives

- to promote active lifestyles

- to provide a safe, climate controlled, well-lit area to walk

- to reinforce/recognize individuals who are active

Materials/Equipment Needed

- log book to track walking distance

- distance wheel (available at home improvement center)

- store map with color coded, measured, walking routes

- large clock with a second hand for pulse measurement

- optional: automatic blood pressure machine

- optional: information kiosk dispensing fitness information

- optional: bulletin board displaying member's success, noteworthy fitness topics/advice

Procedures and Teaching Strategies

- use goals and rewards to encourage regular physical activity

Program Description

This program encourages individuals to be active by providing them with a safe, climate controlled, well-lit environment in which to walk. Participants use a log book to keep track of the distance they have covered. A color-coded map outlines a variety of walking routes through the store. Individuals tally up the distance they cover each session and record that information in the log book along with their pulse and blood pressure. Participants receive a "Moving Targets" t-shirt upon completion of 25 miles of walking. All walking participants qualify for a special monthly drawing. Prizes are donated by various departments throughout the store.

Moving Targets – A Walking Program

Exercise and Your Health

Regular exercise:
- helps reduce high blood pressure
- helps to control diabetes
- helps to control cholesterol levels and reduce lipids (fats) in the blood
- strengthens the heart
- can help motivate smokers to quit smoking
- when weight-bearing, helps to decrease the risk of developing osteoporosis
- can help persons with arthritis move around more easily
- can help you sleep better
- can help your digestive system maintain regularity and prevent constipation

Aerobic exercise is recommended for weight control. Some examples of aerobic activities:
- walking
- swimming
- cross-country skiing
- stationary cycling
- rowing
- jogging

Guidelines for aerobic activity:
- Frequency: 5 times per week
- Intensity: 60% to 85% of your maximum heart rate, or of moderate intensity, which still allows you to talk while exercising
- Duration: 30 to 60 minutes of aerobic activity per session

Our program is actually YOUR program. YOU set your frequency, intensity and duration. We will provide you with a safe, climate controlled, well-lit area to walk. By recording your mileage, blood-pressure and pulse on the log sheets provided, you can keep account of your progress and earn mileage for free give-away items.

Each week, a suggested route will be outlined for you on the map found at the pharmacy counter. We will have your log sheet available at the counter, too, so you can record your progress. Program hours will be during times when the store is less crowded to allow for your freedom of movement.

Hours of Operation:
Monday through Saturday
7:00 AM to 10:00 AM
and
8:00 PM to 11:00 PM

As with ANY exercise program, we recommend you check with your doctor before participating. This is especially true if you are presently under his/her care for pre-existing medical conditions (heart problems, high blood pressure, weight management). We also recommend good, sturdy and comfortable walking shoes and comfortable clothing. Here's to YOUR HEALTH!

Moving Targets

Preparation For Walking

- Please consult your doctor before beginning this or any program of exercise. This is particularly important if you are being treated for heart condition, high blood pressure, or are overweight and considering losing weight.

- Have good, sturdy, comfortable walking shoes to protect your feet and yourself from injuries.

- Always carry water to drink before, during and after exercising.

- Perform 5 minutes of warm-ups and stretches to prepare your body to move. Some examples are arm circles; leg swings; walking alternately on toes, then heels, then toes again; and cat stretches.

- If you are just beginning a walking program, walk 20 minutes at a natural stroll, swinging arms and breathing deeply for the first two weeks. Some soreness may result at first, especially in the shin areas. This should go away after the first two weeks, as your body becomes accustomed to the exercise.

After Walking

Make sure you stretch on completion of your walk to cool down. Hold each stretch for 10 to 20 seconds. Some examples are lower back and hamstring stretches; hip flexes (also called "lunges"); shin/calf stretches, done from a sitting position; and chest stretches (arm placed UP on wall, standing tall, press forearm to wall, then take a step forward while stretching). Repeat on both sides.

Walking is the safest, cheapest and easiest way to stay in shape and to lose weight. Take your time when starting, and have fun. We hope to see LESS of you in the coming months!

LOG SHEET
MOVING TARGETS

Name _____ Physician _____

Date	Time In	Time Out	Distance Walked	Blood Pressure	Pulse

Total Distance Covered _____

If you suffer from a heart condition, high blood pressure, obesity or **any** condition which requires the supervision or treatment by a doctor, we strongly recommend you get approval to begin this and any other exercise program. Your doctor may want to recommend a pace at which you may begin, and to what extent to increase your exertion level. Target cannot be held responsible for any injuries or accidents which may occur during the scheduled hours of the program.

NOTE: For use by program participants to log their activities at home.

Personal Exercise Log

date	exercise mode	warm-up duration	exercise duration	cool-down duration	exercise HR	comments
Sun						
Mon						
Tue						
Wed						
Thu						
Fri						
Sat						

goals for next week:

71

NOTE: Use store map to display measured walking routes.

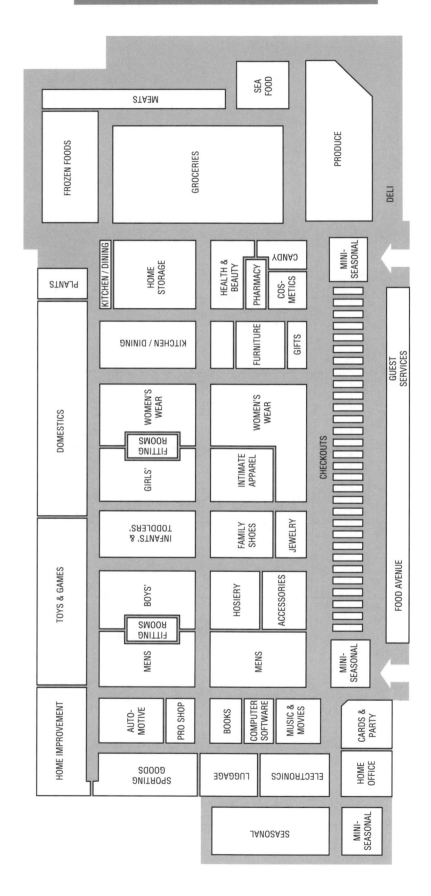

Program Tips

Hold a special monthly incentive drawing in which participants are allowed to fill out an entry form each time they walk. The more they walk, the better their chance of winning.

Plan an awards ceremony to honor all participants as well as top achievers. Challenge participants to continue the "exercise lifestyle."

Contact the media to promote the accomplishments of the participants.

Program graphic could be determined through an art contest.

Feature a month of "buddy" workouts. Encourage participants to adopt a "buddy" and meet with them on a regular basis to walk. For each new participant they bring into the program during this month, award them with double entry forms for incentive drawings.

MOVING TARGETS
ENTRY FORM   DATE _____

NAME _____

ADDRESS _____

CITY _____ STATE _____ ZIP _____

PHONE (_____) _____

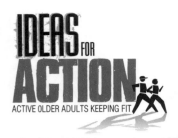

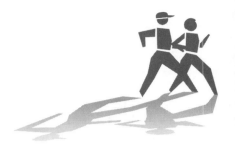

PROGRAM:

Oak Hill Village Fitness Club

Organization: Oak Hill Village
1800 Kensington Drive
Waukesha, WI 53188
Phone: (414) 548-1449
Fax: (414) 548-5981
Contributor: Margaret Finley, Lifestyle Coordinator

Program Description

Developing a Fitness Club for Adults 80+ Living in an Established Retirement Community

The "aging in place" phenomena will eventually challenge every retirement community. A resident's safety and well-being, along with the image the facility portrays to the general community, can be compromised as health and mobility changes of residents affect daily living. Research has shown that regular exercise improves flexibility, strength, endurance, mood and function in older adults. Marketing knows it is much easier to promote a healthy and fit resident population to prospects.

The Laureate Group retirement complex is located in Waukesha, Wisconsin, a community with a population of 60,000, twenty miles west of Milwaukee. It is anchored by Oak Hill Village, with 196 apartments. Residents of this facility live independently. The average age is 82.

The campus is shared with Oak Hill Terrace, which offers assisted living in 175 apartments, Westmoreland Health Center, a 245-bed extended care facility, Omni Home Care and Omni Therapy, a rehabilitation agency.

Program Objectives

In response to the aging in place phenomena, the Laureate Group designed a fitness club to reinforce the value of a pro-active approach to health and wellness. The Village Fitness Club's mission is to provide residents with more comprehensive health monitoring, education services and specialized exercise instruction, to improve general health and well-being, and to help maintain function for as long as possible. The Club provides a setting for established medical services such as a podiatrist and audiologist, as well as technical training and assistance for existing exercise groups.

It was perceived that residents would improve their overall fitness and health, and thereby also improve psychologically and in their ability to care for themselves. The Laureate Group would better meet its mission, improve marketability, decrease resident turnover, generate revenue, and become involved with clinical research. The general community would benefit from the decreased need for medical services.

Materials/Equipment Needed

Following an extensive period of discussions and evaluations, it became evident that inter-company cooperation, with corporate endorsement, would be essential for the Fitness Club to become a reality.

Since the fitness club concept required involvement from Omni Therapy, Oak Hill Village, Omni Home Care and the Laureate Group, the identification of requirements and responsibilities was essential.

Dedicated space was identified and construction and remodeling was undertaken. The Club consists of a small gym and office area. The equipment and supplies needed for the Club are listed below.

- desk and chair
- weight scale
- mats
- exercise bike
- mirrors
- literature rack
- file and folders
- exercise bench
- hand-held weights and therabands
- treadmill
- pedometer and stop watch

Procedures and Teaching Strategies

Fitness Club Start-Up

Omni therapists and therapy aides provide the twice weekly fitness program and have trained Oak Hill Village recreation staff in proper exercise techniques for older adults. The recreation staff holds the new group education and exercise session, as well as continues to educate the existing morning group. Blood pressure screenings and consultation visits with the registered nurse are sponsored by Omni Home Care. In addition, the podiatrist and hearing clinics were moved into the Fitness Club, thus providing privacy for consultations and treatments.

Fitness Club Programs:

Fitness Club Hours: The Club is open 24 hours a day, 7 days a week for independent exercise. This allows residents to use the fitness center according to their lifestyle.

Fitness Evaluations: An Omni Therapy physical therapist completes a fitness assessment and designs exercise recommendations based upon the results of the evaluation and individual resident goals.

Fitness Trainer Sessions: An Omni Therapy Senior Aide is available on Monday and Thursday afternoons for 2 1/2 hours. The trainer assists with equipment orientation, demonstrates proper exercise techniques and provides support and encouragement.

Morning Walk Club: A recreation specialist leads a walk club every Friday morning at 9:30 a.m. The group meets at the Fitness Club and walks throughout the building or at indoor malls in the winter, and on the grounds and at local parks in the summer.

Ask a Nurse: An Omni Home Care registered nurse consults privately on the 1st and 3rd Tuesdays of every month.

Blood Pressure Checks: Held in the Fitness Club weekly.

Podiatrist and Hearing Aid Clinics: All visits from outside specialists are conducted in the Fitness Club.

Educational Opportunities: Seminars and educational talks are scheduled in the Fitness Club.

Program Results

- Currently, 85-90 residents utilize the Fitness Club in one or more programs.

- Therapists and trainers have learned to celebrate and reward small incremental goals, which is a very important technique for keeping participants motivated.

- The Club has distinguished Oak Hill Village from its competition.

- The Fitness Club has received very positive reactions from touring older adults and their families.

Program Tip

- **Design an informational brochure** about your fitness program/facility and distribute to potential users. Include in welcome packets and the monthly community newsletter. Distribute information about new program offerings as it becomes available.

Exercise...the Fountain of Youth!

How would you like to:

- **Feel more relaxed**
- **Lose weight or stop smoking**
- **Enjoy a sense of satisfaction**

- **Have more fun**
- **Be in control of your health**

A recent series of Gallup surveys showed that people who exercise regularly experience all of the above as their strength and energy improve. Added long term health benefits include reducing the risk of hip and wrist fractures.

A three-year study at the USDA Research Center on Aging indicates that seniors who weight-train have at least 100% improvement in leg strength and an average 20% improvement in the time it takes to walk down a hall or up stairs.

You can improve your health and fitness. It isn't easy. It takes work. But it's worth it!

Take Control of Your Health at the Village Fitness Club!

- The Club is equipped with specialized fitness equipment. After proper instruction, you can use the equipment whenever you like. The Club is open for exercise and fitness training seven days a week.

- The Club Trainer will recommend and supervise a personal training program, based on your individual needs to help you increase strength and flexibility.

- At a small group exercise class you can enjoy exercising with others, while working on a personal fitness program recommended just for you.

- Join a new afternoon fitness group called "Fitness Edge." Designed with posture in mind, this class will work on different muscle groups to increase your strength and endurance.

- If you enjoy walking, you'll have fun with "Follow the Leader." This walking group meets weekly and logs their mileage with the help of a pedometer. Sometimes they walk indoors and other times it's to an exciting outdoor destination.

And More....

- Weekly Omni Home Care blood pressure checks will be held in the Fitness Club.

- The podiatrist and hearing specialist will also be scheduled in the Club.

- The Club's registered nurse will be available by appointment to meet with you in the private office to answer any questions you may have and to provide information and referral services for you.

- Monthly socials, lectures and special guests are planned with health and fitness in mind. You can expect special interest groups to form for in-depth conversations about topics like diabetes, arthritis and others.

To Get Started:

- See the Oak Hill Village Lifestyle staff to get started!

- As with any exercise program, we recommend that you check with your physician before beginning.

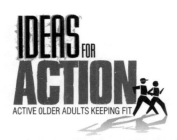

ACTIVE OLDER ADULTS KEEPING FIT

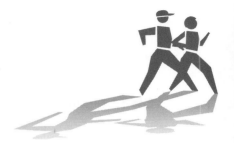

Partners in Fitness, Inc.

Organization:	Partners in Fitness, Inc.
	7 Gibson Avenue
	Dedham, MA 02026
Phone:	(781) 326-6917
Fax:	(781) 326-3107
e-mail:	pifinc@aol.com
Contributor:	Linda Mazie, M.Ed., President

Strength Training Program

Program Objective

- to increase muscle and bone mass

Materials/Equipment Needed

- 3-6 pieces of Keiser equipment (chest press, seated row, lat pulldown, leg press, leg extension, seated leg curl)

- desk with one-sided file drawer and top drawer and chair

- 3 chairs or bench for residents

- water bubbler with cups

- trash can

- cork board

- music box

- hanging file folders and cart

- manila file folders

- 5-10 clipboards

- pens and pencils

- 2-3 stacking trays for top of desk

- 3-ring binder

- 2 wall hanging organizers (one to keep clip boards and one to keep copies of articles)

- 3-6 hooks to hang clipboards next to or on each machine

- 1-2 five pound adjustable ankle weights

- 1-2 sets of each of the following dumbbells – 1, 2, 3, 4 and 5 pounds

- 2-3 sets of dynabands – light, medium and heavy resistance

- Borg Scale of Perceived Exertion wall chart (see page 3)

- 1-2 Rubbermaid foot stools

Procedures and Teaching Strategies

Recommended staffing:

Hours based on size of facility:

Under 100 residents = 6 - 9 hours per week; Over 100 residents = 9 - 20 hours per week.

All hours spread out over 3 times per week.

Staff training options:

- Hire a consultant to design and develop exercise room

- Hire a consultant to operate exercise room

- Hire a consultant to train facility staff to operate exercise room

- Hire facility staff with experience in Strength Training Programming for the older adult

Staff should be trained on how to use the equipment, emergency procedures, benefits of exercise and safety.

Educating the residents:

1. Provide resident orientation on the benefits and importance of exercise.

2. Train each resident individually to:

   - establish safety,

   - explain methods of strength training,

   - establish starting weight and seat adjustment on each machine.

3. Review and circulate physician consent and resident liability forms.

Getting started:

1. Prepare sign-up sheet for initial assessments.

2. Complete exercise room set-up.

3. Prepare sign-up sheet for initial appointments.

4. After the initial appointments, continue the sign-up sheets to schedule workout times and allow 30 minutes per resident. (For example, if you have 6 machines, 6 residents can sign up every 30 minutes. This will allow 24 residents to participate in a 2 hour period. As time goes on, some of the residents will be able to use the equipment independently.)

5. For assisted living facilities with low functioning residents, and residents with Alzheimer's disease, staff will want to schedule one-on-one appointments on an ongoing basis.

Forms needed:

- resident liability

- physician consent

- assessment

- resident files

- exercise logs

- sign-up sheets

Program Description

This is a comprehensive, state of the art strength training program enabling the user to begin at zero pounds of resistance and work up in as little as one pound increments, while feeling safe on the equipment.

Program Results

- builds muscle and increases muscle strength and endurance

- strengthens connective tendons, ligaments and supporting bony structures

- builds power, which is shown to be an important factor in preventing falls in older adults

- increases joint mobility and flexibility

- aids in weight control

- gastrointestinal transit time increases, preventing constipation, diverticulitis, colitis, etc.

- improves posture, balance, coordination, emotional outlook, sleep pattern, physical appearance

- strengthens accident resistance and enhances disease resistance

- enhances self-esteem and alertness, social interaction and independence

- sense of well-being and mood improvement

Program Tips

- **Incorporate exercise room materials (information and forms) in "welcome packets"** so a new resident can have their initial assessment or appointment as they move in.

- When beginning an exercise program in an existing facility, **start with a presentation/Open House** to educate, excite and encourage the residents to participate.

- **Include incentive and motivational programming** in order to successfully market your program.

- **Use pre- and post-assessment success stories** to promote your exercise program.

- **Write articles for the community newsletter about fitness topics** and tie it in to residents' lives.

- **Create an attractive flyer** which tells about your facility/program.

Note: Contact Linda Mazie in regard to consultation services for retirement communities. See *Senior Fitness Consultants* in the *Resource* section.

Rate of Perceived Exertion Scale

6	
7	Very, very light
8	
9	Very light
10	
11	Fairly light
12	
13	Somewhat hard
14	
15	Hard
16	
17	Very hard
18	
19	Very, very hard
20	

Perceived exertion is a method used to monitor exercise intensity. Select a rating that corresponds to your subjective perception of how hard you are exercising when training within your target heart rate zone. As you exercise, you will become familiar with the amount of exertion required to raise your heart rate to your target level by using the Rate of Perceived Exertion Scale.

Strength Training Program Resident Liability Form

Participant's name: _____

The purpose of a Strength Training Program is to improve muscle strength and functional capacity for everyday activities through a progressive personal exercise program. The activities are designed to place a gradually increasing work load on the cardiorespiratory and musculoskeletal systems and thereby improve their function.

I have voluntarily enrolled in a program of progressive physical exercise. I understand that participation in such a program is a potentially hazardous activity, which involves many risks. These risks include but are not limited to: muscle soreness, abnormal blood pressure, fainting, accidents, falling, disorders of heart beat, and in rare instances, heart attack. Obviously, effort will be made to minimize these risks to the individual by preliminary examination and by observation during any situation of which staff is made aware. To my knowledge, I do not have any limiting physical condition or disability which would preclude an exercise program. I and anyone entitled to act on my behalf do thereby release **facility name** and any of their employees or representatives from all claims or liabilities what-so-ever arising from my participation in this program. I agree to assume all risk and responsibility for any injury, damage or other adverse occurrence which may result from my participation in this program.

I understand that a completed physician consent form will be required before I can begin a Strength Training Program. I also understand that each individual may react differently to fitness activities, and that these reactions cannot be predicted with complete accuracy. I understand that I am responsible for informing the fitness staff or my health care professional if I experience any unusual symptoms or if pains should occur. I understand that in the event of an injury, assistance will be readily available and I will not hold the staff of **facility name** responsible for any injuries sustained by me in this program.

Participant's signature: _____ Date:_____

Strength Training Program Physician Consent Form

Participant's Name: _____ Age: _____

Room Number: _____ Telephone: _____

★ ★

Dear Doctor,

Your patient has applied to participate in a Strength Training Program at *facility name*. Upon entering the program, the exercise staff will perform an informal assessment to determine an appropriate exercise program. Tests will be performed to assess strength, endurance, agility and balance. If you have any questions, call *contact person*. You may return this form with your patient or fax to *facility name* at *facility fax number*.

Relevant Medical Conditions: _____

Relevant Medications: _____

Precautions or Recommendations: _____

_____

Please circle YES or NO: **This patient may participate in...**

Yes or No: **Supervised Strength Training Program** (List type of equipment here.)

Yes or No: **Unsupervised Strength Training Program** (List type of equipment here.)

Yes or No: **Supervised use of cardiovascular equipment** (List type of equipment here.)

Yes or No: **Unsupervised use of cardiovascular equipment** (List type of equipment here.)

Additional comments _____

_____

★ ★

Referring Physician (please print): _____ Phone: _____

Address: _____

Physician Signature: _____ Date: _____

Fitness Assessments for Strength Training Program

Program Objective

- to measure balance, endurance, agility, and strength before and after participating in a strength training program

Materials/Equipment Needed

- distance wheel (available at home improvement center)
- stop watch
- tape measure
- 17" high chair
- cone and/or marker
- forms and testing protocol

Procedures and Teaching Strategies

There are a variety of fitness assessments being used throughout the country for studies on strength training and the older adult. The assessments used by *Partners in Fitness, Inc.* are taken from assorted facilities and are based on our experience in ease of testing and data gathering.

Assess prior to beginning the strength training program and reassess after four (4) months of consistent strength training (3 times a week). Testing can continue on a semi-annual basis.

Fitness assessments can be performed for strength training exercise classes as well.

Program Description

Participants sign up for 20 - 30 minute assessments depending on ability range of resident. Explain the tests, reason for testing, benefits of strength training and the goals of strength training three (3) times per week. Document and file the assessment results.

Program Results

Results should show improvement in balance, agility, strength and endurance.

Program Tips

- **Encourage all residents** to participate in fitness assessments, even if assistive devices are used.
- **Use assessment results** to market exercise programs within and outside of your facility.

Note: Contact Linda Mazie in regard to consultation services for retirement communities. See *Senior Fitness Consultants* in the *Resource* section.

Fitness Assessment Protocol

Review and demonstrate to participants all assessments before starting.

Chair Stand

Use chair without arms, 17" high. Begin in the middle of the seat with arms crossed at wrist and held against the chest. Stand up and sit down as many times as possible within 30 seconds.

Timed Up and Go

Use chair 17" high and cone/marker placed 10 feet away from the front of the chair. Record time it takes to get up from the chair to the cone/marker and back to a seated position in the chair.

Balance

Static balance: Stand as they normally do. Let go of any assistive device when they feel ready. Hold for 15 seconds.

Can use arms to balance, but not to physically touch anything.

Parallel foot stance: Begin with feet together and hold this position for 15 seconds.

Tandem stance: Stand with the heel of one foot touching the toes of the other foot. Put either foot forward. Hold for 15 seconds.

One-legged stance: Stand with one foot on the floor and lift the other foot off the floor, using either foot, whichever is more comfortable. Hold for 15 seconds.

Scoring: Maximum score is 15 seconds for all balance tests. Record number of seconds participant was able to hold the balance without needing any assistive devices.

Six (6) Minute Walk

Using a distance wheel to mark feet traveled, begin walking with participant at their pace, with the goal of going the most distance possible within a timed six (6) minute period. Note whether the participant uses an assistive device, or holds on to the tester. Encourage participants to reduce intensity in order to increase duration.

Fitness Assessment for Older Adults

Name_____ Age _____

Pre date _____/_____/_____

Post date _____/_____/_____

Number of exercise sessions between pre & post assessments:_____

	Pre:	Post:
Chair stand:	_____	_____
Method: (circle one)	without arms	without arms
	with arms	with arms
	attempted but unable	attempted but unable
	refused	refused
Comments:		
Timed Up and Go	_____	_____
Assistive device	_____	_____
Comments:		
Balance: (15 seconds max.)		
Static/Normal	_____	_____
Parallel	_____	_____
Tandem	_____	_____
One-legged	_____	_____
Comments:		
Six (6) minute walk:		
Distance traveled	_____	_____
Assistive device	_____	_____
Comments:		

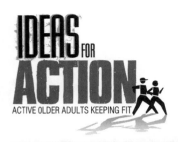

IDEAS FOR ACTION

ACTIVE OLDER ADULTS KEEPING FIT

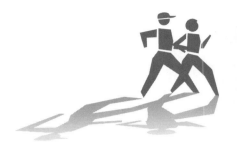

Plano Senior Games

Organization:	City of Plano Senior Center
	401 West 16th Street
	P.O. Box 860358
	Plano, TX 75086-0358
Phone:	(972) 461-7155
Fax:	(972) 461-7415
Contributor:	Dell Kaplan

Plano Senior Games is based on the State Games and Senior Games concept. Activities offered are dictated in part by the facilities a community has available, as well as the interests of potential participants.

Program Objectives

- to provide an opportunity for persons age 50 years or older to participate in organized sports activities

- to promote activity as an integral part of a "well" lifestyle

Materials/Equipment Needed

- equipment and venue sites for the chosen activities

- promotional piece which includes information on the "Games"

- registration form

Program Description

The Plano Senior Games have been in existence for 10 years. A wide variety of sports and participation-type events are held over a two-week period. The "Games" start with a kick-off breakfast, and an awards dinner dance is held upon completion.

Program Tips

- **Promote Senior Games** not only to Senior Center participants, but display information about the games in grocery stores, physician's offices, public informational kiosks, malls, etc.

- **Include a mix of non-sport recreational activities** in order to appeal to a wider range of participants. By involving these individuals in a non-sport activity, they may be motivated to become active in order to participate in a sport activity in future "Games."

PLANO SENIOR GAMES
MARCH 10 - 21

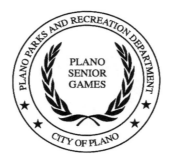

ELIGIBILITY: Any person 50 years or older as of March 10, who is currently an amateur in the event for which he/she registers, is eligible to participate.

AGE GROUPS: Age and sex divisions will be determined by Events Committee as registration requires. There must be a minimum of three registered participants in an event for it to take place.

REGISTRATION DEADLINE: All entries must be returned or postmarked no later than March 6 with the exception of Duplicate Bridge, March 3. The Liability Waiver must be signed and accompany your registration. A $5.00 non-refundable registration fee must accompany each form. Please do not mail cash. Send entries to: PLANO SENIOR GAMES, P.O. BOX 860358, PLANO, TEXAS 75086-0358.

REGISTRATION FEE: A $5.00 fee entitles you to participate in as many events as you desire and admission to the Opening Breakfast. Some events, such as bowling, golf and miniature golf require an additional facility fee.

AWARDS: First place medals may be picked up at the Awards Banquet. Ribbons not distributed at events may be picked up at the Senior Center after March 21.

OPENING BREAKFAST: The Games will begin with a Kick-Off Breakfast at Plano Centre at 8:30 a.m. on March 10th. All participants will be admitted free. Price for guests is $5.50, non-refundable. Please RSVP when you register.

AWARDS DINNER DANCE: March 21st, Harvey Hotel, Plano, 6 - 9 p.m., doors open at 5:30 p.m. Tickets are $10.50 for participants at registration, $16.50 for non-participating spouse or guest.

CANCELLATIONS: In the event of inclement weather or unusual circumstances, Games officials reserve the right to cancel or postpone events to a later time. Officials reserve the right to reschedule, cancel or change event times based on registration.

REGISTRATION BEGINS FEBRUARY 1ST
For more information call 972-461-7155

TIP: Enlarge type to make registration information easier to read.

SCHEDULE OF EVENTS

MONDAY, MARCH 10

Kick-Off Breakfast	8:30 am	Plano Centre, 2000 E. Sprint Creek Pky.
Goofy Games	10:30 am	Plano Senior Center
Bridge (Duplicate)	1:00 pm	Plano Senior Center
Track & Field	12:00 noon	Williams High School, 1712 Ave. P

TUESDAY, MARCH 11

Basketball Shoot	8:30 am	Plano Rec. Center, 701 Coit at Legacy
Billiards - Women's	9:30 am	Plano Senior Center

WEDNESDAY, MARCH 12

Billiards - Men	9:00 am	Plano Senior Center
Swimming & Water Fitness	10:00 am	Aquatic Center, 2301 Westside Dr.
Table Tennis	3-5 pm	Plano Senior Center

THURSDAY, MARCH 13

Golf - Men (Raindate 3/20)	8:30 am	Pecan Hollow Golf Course, 4501 E. 14th St.
Golf - Women (Raindate 3/20)	8:30 am	Pecan Hollow Golf Course
Line Dance & Tap Dance Party	1:00 pm	Plano Senior Center

FRIDAY, MARCH 14

Croquet	9:30 am	Plano Senior Center
Open Bridge (Singles)	1:00 pm	Plano Senior Center
Pinochle	1:00 pm	Plano Senior Center
"42"	1:00 pm	Plano Senior Center

MONDAY, MARCH 17

Bridge (Pairs)	1:00 pm	Plano Senior Center

TUESDAY, MARCH 18

Checkers	8:30 am	Plano Senior Center
Skipbo, Dominoes	10:00 am	Plano Senior Center
Walking	10:00 am	Sunny Day, Plano Senior Center
		Rainy Day, Plano Recreation Center
Gin Rummy	1:00 pm	Plano Senior Center

WEDNESDAY, MARCH 19

Bowling - Men's	9:30 am	Plano Super Bowl
Bowling - Women's	1:00 pm	Plano Super Bowl

THURSDAY, MARCH 20

Arts & Crafts	9 am - 1 pm	Public invited from noon to 1 pm, Plano Senior Center
Bocce Ball	9:00 am	Plano Senior Center
Miniature Golf	2:00 pm	Mountasia Fantasy, 900 Premier Drive

FRIDAY, MARCH 21

Horseshoes	9:00 am	Plano Senior Center
Baking Judging starts	10:00 am	Plano Senior Center
Awards Dinner Dance	6 - 9 pm	Harvey Hotel, 1600 No. Central, Doors open at 5:30 pm

S A M P L E   H A N D O U T

TIP: When reproducing for handouts, copy pages 90 and 91 back to back. Enlarge type to make registration information easier to read.

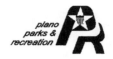

PLANO SENIOR GAMES REGISTRATION FORM

Please complete both sides of this registration form and include all fees. Each individual must enter on a separate form. When selecting events, please check the Event Schedule to avoid time conflicts. **Return this page.** Mark your events on the Event Schedule and retain.

If paying by check, please make it payable to **Plano Senior Games** and mail to:

> Plano Senior Center
> P.O. Box 860358
> Plano, TX 75086-0358

PLEASE TYPE OR PRINT

NAME_____ BIRTHDATE _____

ADDRESS_____ SEX   M (   ) F (   )

CITY _____ STATE _____ ZIP _____

TELEPHONE Home (_____) _____ Other (_____) _____

REGISTRATION DEADLINE IS MARCH 6
DUPLICATE BRIDGE, MARCH 3

THE PLANO SENIOR GAMES RECOMMENDS THAT PARTICIPANTS CONSULT THEIR PHYSICIAN IN REGARD TO PRACTICE, PREPARATION AND COMPETITION IN THE PLANO SENIOR GAMES.

PERTINENT MEDICAL INFORMATION (medical condition, special medication, allergies, other information): Please attach any additional information necessary to ensure your health and safety.

EMERGENCY CONTACT:

Name _____

Relationship _____ Phone _____

LIABILITY WAIVER

I, the undersigned participant, hereby agree to indemnify, save and hold harmless the Plano Senior Games, Plano Parks & Recreation Department and the City of Plano, any site associated with Plano Senior Games, or any of its agents or representatives. I have prepared myself for the events which I have entered by practicing prior to this Senior Games. To the best of my knowledge and belief, I have no physical restrictions which would prohibit my participation in the events I have selected. I, the undersigned participant, grant to the Plano Senior Games the right to use any pictures taken of me during the Plano Senior Games to be held March 10 through March 21, inclusive, 1997 without my remuneration.

Signature _____ Date _____

TIP: When reproducing for handouts, copy pages 90 and 91 p back to back. Enlarge type to make registration information easier to read.

EVENT REGISTRATION

Registration fee of $5.00 covers as many events as you wish to enter. (Some events require a facility usage fee.) **Please check your choices:**

ARTS & CRAFTS _____
    Category _____
BAKING _____
    Category _____
BASKETBALL SHOOT _____
BILLIARDS _____
    Men _____ Women _____
BOCCE BALL _____
BOWLING _____
    Men _____ Women _____
    Average _____
BRIDGE
    Singles (3/14) _____
    Pairs (3/17) _____
    Your Partner's name _____
    Duplicate (3/10) _____
    Your Partner's name _____
CARD GAMES
    Gin Rummy _____
    Skipbo _____
    Pinochle _____
CROQUET _____
DANCE EXHIBITION
    Line Dance _____
    Tap _____
GOLF
    Men _____
    Women _____
    Open _____
    Handicap _____ Ride _____ Walk _____

GOOFY GAMES _____
HORSESHOES _____
MINIATURE GOLF _____
SWIM MEET
    25 m Backstroke _____
    50 m Backstroke _____
    Underwater _____
    25 m Freestyle _____
    50 m Freestyle _____
    25 m Water Walk _____
    25 m Breaststroke _____
    50 m Breaststroke _____
    Other _____
    Water Exercises _____
TABLE GAMES
    Checkers _____
    Dominoes _____
    "42" _____
TABLE TENNIS
    Men _____
    Women _____
TRACK & FIELD
    50 m Dash _____
    100 m Dash _____
    Discus _____
    Shot Put_____
    Long Jump _____
    Other _____
WALKING
    1 Mile _____
    3 Mile _____

I HAVE ENCLOSED:

REGISTRATION FEE $ _____5.00
OPENING BREAKFAST – I will attend _____   _____-0-
    Breakfast Guests at $5.50 each   _____
AWARDS DINNER
    Participant @ $10.50   _____
    Dinner guests @ $16.50 each   _____
TOTAL FEES: $ _____

PLANO PARKS AND RECREATION DEPARTMENT
PLANO SENIOR GAMES
CITY OF PLANO

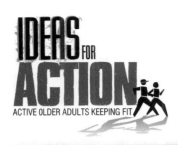

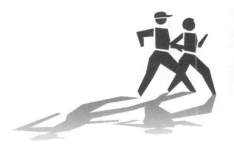

PROGRAM:

S.E.E. S.A.W. Exercises
Seniors Exercising Effectively While Sitting Around Waiting

Organization: SENioRS Unlimited
(Senior Exercise Networks Resources & Services)
7880 Fowler Lane
Bozeman, MT 59718
Phone: (406) 587-0786
e-mail: Kayvn@montana.campus.mci.net
Contributor: Kay Van Norman, President

Program Objectives

- to empower Seniors to take an active role in maintaining their physical function regardless of level of functional ability

- to integrate functional movement training throughout their daily lives by teaching them that all "Movement Matters"

- to focus on movements that will help Seniors maintain the ability to perform the activities of daily living (frail seniors)

- to encourage proper body alignment and movement patterns, and reinforce the concept of how repetitive movement patterns can have a positive or negative effect on maintaining functional ability over a lifetime (active seniors)

Materials/Equipment Needed

- brochures that illustrate a series of exercises and can be used by the individual seniors, or posters placed on the wall

- ankle weights are optional – can be used by a participant going through the whole exercise brochure

Procedures and Teaching Strategies

Seniors are provided with an exercise brochure and a set of weights that are adjustable from 1-5 pounds.

They then are instructed that many of the exercises can be done at any time while they are "sitting around waiting" for something. For example: ankle flexions and toe curls, knee lifts or extensions, hand mobility, finger stretch, cross arm, elbow lift, bicep curl, shoulder press. Encourage them to do the exercises as many times a day as possible (without weights).

Participants are encouraged to perform the brochure program at home with weights 3-4 days per week, starting with the minimum number of repetitions and progressing over time to the maximum number of repetitions.

Have them increase the weight when they can easily lift the lower weight the maximum number of repetitions.

Program Description

Many frail seniors have to sit waiting for rides, waiting for meals if in a group facility, etc. This is a great time to work on functional ability. Even in public, many of the exercises can be done "undetected."

Program Results

It has inspired many people to move who otherwise would not take the time to attend an exercise class.

In a senior residence facility with 62 residents, only 18-20 regularly attended the chair exercise class. However, when given the opportunity to follow an exercise brochure/program in their own apartment, 48 asked to receive the information.

Program Tip

- **Customize the exercises** to address the various needs of the participants.

Program Note:

Note: Contact Kay Van Norman in regard to consultation services for retirement communities. See *Senior Fitness Consultants* in the *Resource* section. To purchase exercise brochures, contact Kay Van Norman at (406) 587-0786.

YOU <u>CAN</u> MAKE A DIFFERENCE !!

Numerous studies have proven that increased physical activity can have a significant effect on maintaining and improving your physical function. It is clear that disuse invites decay. Decay invites dependence. Increasing your physical activity is a GREAT way to take an active role in maintaining your independence and thus your quality of life! This simple program is designed to help you maintain strength, mobility, coordination and balance.

You will need approximately 15 minutes, a chair with no arms which allows you to sit forward comfortably with your feet flat on the floor, and one set of ankle weights (2 1/2 pounds each). Please contact your instructor if you have difficulty finding appropriate weights.

The warm-up/coordination exercises should be performed at a moderate tempo, swinging the arms freely. Loss of coordination occurs rapidly if a person does not engage in activities which require performing coordinated patterns. The objective of this segment is to warm up the joints of the body, challenge your coordination (don't be discouraged if opposition is difficult at first), and have some fun. Experiment freely with arms swinging in opposition, and in unison (same arm forward as leg), as well as adding completely different arm movements such as pushing the palms overhead, out to the side, straight out to the front, etc. Using music you enjoy can also add some motivation!

The "elevator" exercise helps maintain the leg function necessary for rising from a chair. Another fun variation is the use of a rhyme where you "act out" some of the words. "The Noble Duke of York, he had 10,000 men, he marched them (up) the hill and marched them (down) again. When they were (up) they were up, and when they were (down) they were down, and when they were only halfway up, they were neither (up) nor (down). Each time "up" occurs in parentheses, stand up, and each time "down" occurs in parentheses, sit back down. At the phrase "when they were only halfway up," stand in a crouched position, knees slightly bent, straightening the knees fully only at the next "up."

The balance segment is designed to help you practice and challenge your balance. The loss of balance resulting in increased falls is of great concern to many older adults. Studies document that the gradual loss of strength and mobility, as well as lack of confidence in balance, strongly influence the likelihood of falls. Research also shows that balance can be regained with practice! Please begin with caution. Do not lean heavily on the chairback, as this could result in the chair falling over backwards. Use good posture – don't look down.

You will receive the most benefit if you perform the balance exercises in stocking or bare feet which allow the feet and toes to move freely. Be cautious of slippery flooring if you are in stocking feet.

When you have mastered each of the balance activities you may increase the time spent in the "balanced" phase of the exercise and/or you may change your arm position. For example, in the knee lift you may begin with the hands resting on the chair, then lift them slightly from the chair, then progress to raising them out-stretched to the sides. A variation of the heel/toes walks can easily be performed down a hallway with your hand resting on the wall as you progress forward and backward. Proceed slowly, mastering each exercise for several weeks before progressing to more difficult variations.

Don't underestimate the importance of the Achilles stretch and the ankle flexion/toe curls. The loss of mobility in the ankle, weakness in the front of the leg (shin), tightness in the back of the leg (calf) and mobility of the feet and toes contributes significantly to falls. The ankle flexion/toe curls is a great exercise to do anytime you find yourself sitting around waiting for something, watching TV, reading, etc.; the more the better!

Strength and mobility of the hips, knees, ankles, shoulders, wrists and hands are all important factors in maintaining the ability for self-care, identified by the medical profession as Basic Activities of Daily Living (BADL's). The strength exercises are designed to be performed with a set of soft ankle weights. An ankle weight can be held in the hand for the upper body exercises or strapped to the ankle for the lower body exercises. If you can easily perform the strength exercises with 2-1/2 pounds and prefer to use more weight, you may use both ankle weights on one leg (for a total of 5 pounds) while performing the seated knee lifts and the knee extensions. However, with both weights on one leg, rather than alternating legs, perform a full exercise sequence on one leg (for example, left knee lift 4-8 times, then left knee extension and hold 4-8 times; then repeat the sequence with the weights on the right leg).

Finally, if you are over the age of 40, you should consult with your physician before beginning any exercise program. If you begin to feel dizzy or fatigued, or experience pain, you should discontinue the program and consult your physician.

Kay has a masters degree in Physical Education/Health and is the former director of "Young at Heart," an exercise program for senior citizens based at Montana State University. She is also the author of "Exercise Programming for Older Adults," published by Human Kinetics Publishers. Contact Kay at (406) 587-0786 with comments, questions, or to order brochures.

MOVEMENT MATTERS!!!
HOME BASED EXERCISE PROGRAM
MAINTAINING INDEPENDENCE THROUGH MOVEMENT

WARM-UP / COORDINATION

These exercises should be performed in *neutral forward position*: seated slightly forward in the chair, back straight, shoulders and arms relaxed. Choose a chair that has a firm seat and back, no arms, and is high enough so your feet comfortably touch the floor when seated.

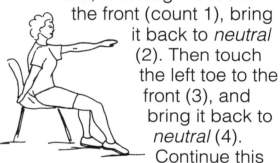

♥ Toe Touch: Extend the right foot forward, touching the toe to the front (count 1), bring it back to *neutral* (2). Then touch the left toe to the front (3), and bring it back to *neutral* (4). Continue this pattern for 16 counts. The arms can swing naturally (one forward, one backward), in opposition – when the right leg is forward, the left arm swings forward.

♥ Heel Press: Repeat the same sequence described in toe touches except instead of touching with the toes, press the heel out with the foot flexed.

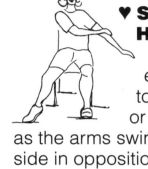

♥ Side Toe Touch / Heel Press: Repeat these exercises, touching the toe or heel side to side as the arms swing from side to side in opposition (as shown).

♥ Elevator: Begin with the feet a comfortable distance apart and arms relaxed at your sides. Stand up slowly by imagining you are an elevator rising 3 floors, stopping briefly (by holding your position for a slow 2 count – 1001, 1002 – at each "floor"). Don't hold your breath! Return to a seated position, making the same "stops" at each position.

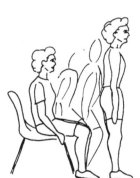

BALANCE

If possible, balance exercises should be done in stocking or bare feet to allow your feet and toes to work freely. Use caution and bare feet if the flooring is slick. Begin by standing behind the chair in *neutral position*; feet a comfortable distance apart with toes pointing straight forward, back straight, shoulders relaxed and hands resting *lightly* on the back of the chair. Do not grip the chairback or lean forward onto the chair.

♥ **Knee Lift Balance:** Lift the right knee up until the foot is off the ground and the lower leg hangs loosely. Hold this position for a slow 4 count, then return to *neutral position*. Repeat with the left leg. Repeat 4 times on each leg. Become aware of feeling your balance without relying on the chair. With practice you may progress to holding the balanced position longer (8-12 counts), and when this is mastered, you may also try the exercise with the hands held slightly off of the chair. Keep an upright posture! Breathe!

♥ **Knee Bends / Tip Toes:** Slowly bend the knees, keeping them in a direct line over the toes (count 1-4 bending), then straighten the legs (count 5-8). Now, with straight legs, raise to the toes and hold this position (1-4), return to *neutral* (5-8). Repeat the full sequence 4-8 times. When you feel more confident, you may progress to lifting your hands slightly off of the chair while balancing on your toes.

♥ **Heel to Toe Walks:** Stand in an upright posture behind the chair with the right hand resting lightly on the corner of the chairback, eyes focused forward (not down). Begin walking forward by placing the heel of one foot *directly* in front of the other (heel touching the toe). Your hand should slide along the top of the chairback. Walk as far as you

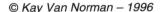

can while still maintaining an upright posture and contact with the chair. Return to the starting position by repeating the same heel to toe walk backwards. Repeat walking forward, then backward 4 times. Then turn to the other side so the left hand is resting on the chair and repeat the full sequence.

♥ **Achilles Stretch:** Standing behind the chair in a left-leg-forward lunge position (forward foot flat on the floor, knee bent), press the right heel toward the floor (right leg straight), hold for a slow count of 16. Return to *neutral*. Repeat on the opposite side in right-leg-forward lunge position.

♥ **Ankle Flexion / Toe Curls:** Seated in *neutral-back position* (scooted back in chair, with back straight but resting on the chairback). Flex the ankles as far

as possible while keeping the heels on the floor. Hold for 8 counts. Relax feet to *neutral,* then curl the toes under (4 counts), flex toes up and wiggle them freely (8 counts), relax to *neutral*. Repeat full sequence 4-8 times beginning with ankle flexion.

STRENGTH / MOBILITY

The strength exercises use a set of soft ankle/wrist weights (each weight is 2 1/2 pounds). Begin seated in the *neutral back position* as described above.

♥ **Knee Lifts:** Place the weights around the ankles. Slowly bring the knee towards the chest as far as possible, while keeping your back straight (count 1-2). Return to *neutral* (3-4). Repeat with the other leg (up 5-6, down 7-8). Repeat full sequence 4-8 times.

♥ **Knee Extensions:** Extend your leg to the front and hold for 8 counts, then bend the knee to return to *neutral*. Repeat the exercise with the other leg. Repeat 4-8 times with each leg. While performing this exercise, extend only through the pain-free range of motion.

♥ **Reach & Squeeze:** Seated slightly forward in the chair with the back straight and shoulders relaxed, extend both arms forward at shoulder level – palms down (count 1-2). Now, keeping elbows up and out to sides (as if using a rolling pin), slowly pull the elbows back by squeezing the shoulder blades together (3-4). Hold (5-8). Repeat 4 to 8 times. Breathe normally! When you become stronger you can do this exercise with the weights held in your hands.

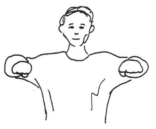

♥ **Hand Mobility:** Seated in a relaxed position, bring your hands up to shoulder level with palms facing forward. Slowly make a fist and then open to beginning position. Repeat 4 times. Now spread the fingers wide open and close 4 times. Then relax the arms to the sides and shake the hands loosely. Repeat entire sequence 4-8 times.

♥ **Finger Stretch:** Rest the hands, palms down, on top of the legs. Using the left hand, gently lift the first finger of the right hand to a stretched position and hold for 8 counts, then release. Repeat with each finger and the thumb. Release the right arm to the side and shake the hand gently. Repeat the full sequence stretching the fingers of the left hand.

The following exercises begin in the neutral forward position; seated slightly forward in the chair with the back straight, the feet flat on the floor, and the arms relaxed at the sides.

♥ **Shoulder Press:** Holding a weight in each hand, bend the elbows and place the hands at shoulder level (palms facing in toward body). Slowly press the weights straight overhead. Slowly return the weights to shoulder level. Repeat this sequence 8-12 times. Breathe normally.

♥ **Biceps Curl:** Still holding a weight in each hand, begin with the arms hanging relaxed at the sides, palms facing toward body. Slowly flex the elbows to bring the hands to the shoulders, then return the arms to the sides in a slow controlled manner. Repeat the sequence 8-12 times.

♥ **Cross Arm:** With empty hands, reach your right arm across the front of your chest to the left. Hold the right forearm with the left hand and gently stretch the right shoulder for a slow 8-16 count. Release the arm opening it around to the front and returning to *neutral* (4 count). Repeat the stretch with the left arm crossing the chest to the right. Repeat 4 times each arm.

♥ **Elbow Lift:** With empty hands, place the right palm on the back of the right shoulder blade. Now slowly raise the right elbow as far as you can, supporting the elbow with the left hand and gently pressing upwards to a stretched position. Hold for 4-8 counts. Maintain an upright posture. Breathe! Release the elbow, bringing the right arm down to the side, shaking gently. Repeat on the left, raising the left elbow and assisting with the right hand. Repeat the entire sequence 4 times.

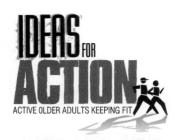

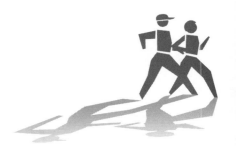

PROGRAM:

Silver Sneakers®

Organization: Court House Plus
Community Fitness & Wellness Center
47 Hartford Turnpike
Vernon, CT 06066
Phone: (860) 649-0597
Fax: (860) 649-3644
Contributor: Jamie Fairley

Program Objective

• to help people take responsibility for their own health

Program Description

Helping people take responsibility for their physical and mental well-being is what the **Silver Sneakers – An Older Adult Fitness Association** is all about. This recreational, social, educational and fitness program is specifically designed for the lifestyle of the 50-plus age group. Courses are offered for fun, fitness and educational fulfillment, and are available to Court House Plus members and non-members alike. "Becoming physically fit is attainable no matter what your age," claims program director, Edna Schuetz.

The following newsletter outlines the Silver Sneakers program offerings.

SILVER SNEAKERS®
An Older Adult Fitness Association

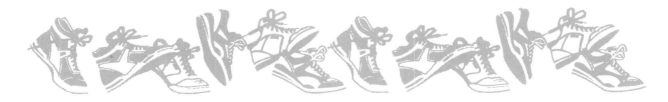

Open House

Tuesday, September 2, 1997
3:30 to 8 p.m.
FREE ADMISSION

Featuring guest appearance of Congresswoman, Barbara Kennelly!

A brief program of class demonstrations will begin at approximately 4 pm. This will be followed by an address on "Health Care for the Older Adult" by Congresswoman, Barbara Kennelly. Everyone is welcome to join us for a delightful buffet in Poolside Cafe. There will be prizes, surprises and drawings. Registration for classes will be taken at the Front Desk. Our evening will conclude with ballroom dancing.

Bring friends and spouses to learn more about the Silver Sneakers program.

Upcoming Trips

A GOLDEN OCTOBERFEST
Wednesday, October 15, 1997

Join the "Silver Sneakers" on a one-day, fun-filled trip featuring Live and Lively entertainment, Hearty Food, Dancing, Merry-making and singing at famous Platzl Brauhaus in upper New York.

BERMUDA
May 2, 1998

You only live once, but if you live right, once is enough! Join us on this relaxing trip to one of the world's most beautiful islands. Experience the culture, the dining extravaganza and many recreational activities. Travel on the ship "Dreamward" – Norwegian Cruiseline's deluxe cruise ship!

SEPTEMBER 11 – 1:30 pm – Thursday – Studio 2: A representative from Collette Travel will give a slide presentation of the Bermuda Cruise. You'll see slides of many points of interest. Bring a friend and enjoy the spectacular show. Question/Answer period to follow.

Fitness Corner

According to the Walking Handbook by Susan Johnson, walking can strengthen your heart, reducing the risk of heart disease and stroke. Just because you're retired doesn't mean you're tired. Maintain your health and level of activity by enrolling in any of the fun Silver Sneakers programs. "You walk every morning, you're active in your community and you're not ready to slow down!"

Wellness Walk with Curly Perzel

Blazing foliage, crisp air, blue sky and a walk in the woods. Trail extends from Valley Falls into Shenipsit Lake trail. Join us in a spaced walk, a comfortable distance from home into a more quiet corner of our world and experience the adventure and challenge of hiking. Always bring water. This hike is for everyone.

Wednesday, Sept. 24th, 9 am
Meet at Court House Plus
Rain Date: October 17th
Fee: $3 (snacks provided)
Call 649-0597 to register.

Soapstone Mountain Hike

Enjoy a foliage hike around and up Soapstone Mountain along the Shenipsit Trail in Somers. We will enjoy a snack and water at the picnic tables near the summit. The hike will be geared to the energy of the group. Distance 4 to 5 miles. Panoramic views. Bring your binoculars.

Wednesday, Oct. 8th, 9 am
Meet at Court House Plus
Rain Date: October 17th
Fee: $3 (snacks provided)
Call 649-0597 to register.

Program Descriptions

Fall classes run for 12 weeks and are FREE to Court House Plus members (unless otherwise noted). Call us at 649-0597. Fees are indicated for non-members. Please make checks payable to COURT HOUSE PLUS.

COUNTRY WESTERN DANCING –

Have fun, meet new people and get some exercise at the same time! Learn the steps of the dances that are sweeping the country and being enjoyed by just plain folks! This is a line dance format – no partner needed and no previous dance experience is necessary.

Tues: noon - 1:30 pm

LINE DANCING –
Line dance is a freestyle of expression through rhythmic body movements done to music. It teaches good posture, coordination, flexibility and improves physical appearance. Wear light-weight leather soled shoes.

Beginner - Tues: 1 - 2:30 pm
Intermediate - Thur: noon - 1:30 pm

GENTLE AEROBICS –
This class is designed to improve overall performance. Low impact aerobics, muscular strengthening exercises and a relaxing stretch will be used to achieve aerobic and muscular conditioning, as well as improved flexibility. Wear comfortable clothing, sneakers and a big smile. Beginners encouraged to attend.

Mon/Wed: 11 am - noon

GENTLE WET WORKOUT –
Learn how to exercise safely in the water while having fun and enjoying the benefits of a great workout. The class will last one hour and will introduce you to both cardiovascular and muscle conditioning exercises in the pool. No swimming experience is necessary.

Tues/Thur: 1:30 - 2:30 pm

OPEN SWIM –
Use the indoor heated pool for laps or relaxation, or to participate in the Aqua Parcourse, an individualized exercise program consisting of 12 exercises which allow you to work at your own fitness level.

Mon/Wed/Fri: 11:30 - 1 pm **or**
Wed/Fri/Sun: 5 - 7:30 pm

STRENGTH TRAINING FOR THE OLDER ADULT –
If you're looking to lower your body fat percentage, blood pressure and cholesterol, have stronger bones, decrease arthritic pain or enjoy many other health benefits, a strength training program could be just the thing you need to improve the quality of your life. Class size is limited to allow for individualized instruction. Have fun while learning some great exercises!

Tues/Thur: 11 am - noon
This is an exceptional value when compared to 1-on-1 personal training fees!

Program Descriptions

TAI CHI CH'UAN Beginner Class –

Tai Chi is an ancient discipline of meditative movements that builds muscle strength, improves balance and relieves stress.

Fri: 9:30 - 10:30 am

TAI CHI CH'UAN for Health & Regeneration – Intermediate Class –

The slow and even movements of Tai Chi Ch'uan relax the body and mind, promoting the flow of vital energy to replace stiffness with flexibility and good body coordination. It promotes mental tranquility, improves physical fitness and increases blood circulation. Most recently, the National Arthritis Foundation has come out in favor of Tai Chi as a suitable exercise for patients afflicted with various forms of disease to ease pain and promote health in the joints.

Wed: Intermediate 10:00 - 11:00 am
Prerequisite: Beginner Class

TAI CHI CH'UAN Advanced Class –

This course is a continuation of intermediate Tai Chi. The emphasis will be on stance and breathing techniques. You will learn the complete form of Tai Chi. The slow relaxed movement and breathing methods will help stimulate the mind and build the body. Please wear comfortable clothing.

Wed: 11:15 am - 12:15 pm
Prerequisite: Beginner &
           Intermediate Class

YOGA – For both beginners and those who have had some instruction in Hatha Yoga postures and breathing. Increases strength, flexibility, and vigor and improves overall physical condition. Wear comfortable exercise wear.

Fri: 11 am - noon

Evening Classes

BALLROOM DANCING – Anyone can learn the foxtrot, waltz, lindy and the macarena in this fun, relaxed course. Although single registrations are accepted, it is recommended that you register with a partner.

Wed: 6:30 - 8 pm
Two sessions of 6 weeks each.

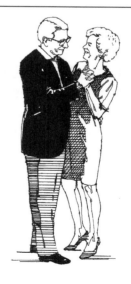

Upcoming Events

All programs are free admission, unless otherwise noted, and require advance registration by calling 649-0597 or visiting Court House Plus.

Wed. Sept. 17 – *WHAT IS A CATARACT*

Our presenter speaks out on what a cataract is, the symptoms and who generally gets them. He will also discuss his invention of "no-stitch" surgery, as well as the procedure's simplicity. A question/answer period will follow.

1:30 pm, Poolside Cafe
Pre-Registration Requested

Tues. Sept. 30 – *LUNGS AT WORK*

This lecture goes beyond the usual inhale-exhale. The speaker will discuss what differentiates diseases such as asthma, emphysema and bronchitis. He will answer questions such as: Besides not smoking, what can be done to take care of our lungs? What happens to our lungs as we grow older?

1:30 pm, Poolside Cafe
Pre-Registration Requested

Thur. Oct. 23 – *EXERCISE FOR PEOPLE WITH ARTHRITIS*

By conservative estimates, half of all seniors suffer from arthritis, leaving many with considerable limitations in their everyday activities. With a few adjustments in lifestyle and treatment as necessary, arthritis need not mean the end of an active, involved outlook on life. The presenter will address all these issues in his presentation on arthritis and reconstructive surgery.

1:30 pm, Poolside Cafe
Pre-Registration Requested

Tues. Oct. 28 – *CLASSICAL GREEK MYTHOLOGY*

The presenter will present a slide lecture on Classical Greek Mythology and Culture. The presentation will take about an hour and a question/answer period will follow.

1:30 pm, Studio 2 - downstairs
Pre-Registration Requested

Thurs. Nov. 13 – *WHY WE FALL*

The presenter will discuss how the eyes, along with the body's ability to sense muscle tension and gravity, are coordinated by the brain to maintain balance.

1:30 pm, Poolside Cafe
Pre-Registration Requested

Wed. Nov. 19 – *EXERCISE, FITNESS & HEALTH*

A program on the impact of exercise and physical fitness on your state of health. We will look at exercise routines, fitness principles and physical changes in your body that result from staying active. Issues such as frequency of exercise, duration of exercise, heart rate, recovery rate and pulse rate will be included in the topics of discussion.

10:30 pm, Poolside Cafe
Pre-Registration Requested

Upcoming Events

Wed. Dec 3 – *ANTIOXIDANTS & FREE RADICALS*

What are they? Come to this informative class and learn how to protect yourself from heart disease and certain types of cancer.

1:30 pm, Poolside Cafe
Pre-Registration Requested

Tues. Dec 10 – *FIBROMYALGIA*

What is Fibromyalgia? Who is affected? Learn signs, symptoms and treatment options for this debilitating condition.

3 pm, Poolside Cafe
Pre-Registration Requested

Wed. Dec 17 – *HOLIDAY PARTY*

Court House Plus members, friends and spouses are invited to attend our annual Silver Sneaker holiday party. A catered lunch will be served, followed by class demonstrations and ballroom dancing. Registrations for winter classes will be taken at the front desk. Be sure to reserve your space for a favorite class or two.

Noon to 4 pm,
Studio 2
Tickets available at the
Front Desk - $12

Friday Night "Live" Ballroom Dancing

Join us for an evening of ballroom dancing with Rae and Del Brigham on the last Friday of every month. Have fun, make new friends and benefit from regular activity. Open to the public. Refreshments available during break time in Poolside Cafe. 7 to 10 pm

DATES: 9/26, 10/31, 11/28
$5 Per Person

Also, see Walking, Hiking and Trip Dates on page two! Keep your eyes open for Square Dancing dates!

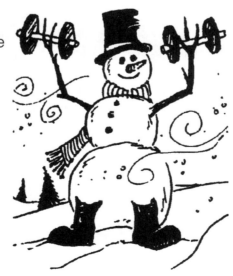

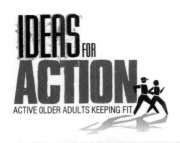

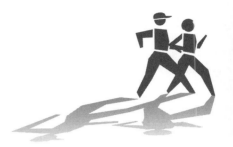

IDEAS FOR ACTION
ACTIVE OLDER ADULTS KEEPING FIT

The Village at Duxbury

Organization:	The Village at Duxbury
	290 Kings Town Way
	Duxbury, MA 02332
Phone:	(781) 585-2334
Fax:	(781) 582-2274
Contributor:	Bonnie Armstrong, Fitness Coordinator

Program Objectives

- to keep residents functioning at a level where they can enjoy life

- to improve posture, flexibility, balance and increase muscle strength and endurance

Materials/Equipment Needed

- appropriate music
- tape player
- resistive machines
- dynabands
- hand-held weights
- towels (alternative to bands)
- pool equipment – resistance gloves, aqua weights, noodles

Procedures and Teaching Strategies

Keep in mind the health issues of the clients. Be familiar with safety precautions during exercise sessions. Be aware that there are special conditions (i.e., advanced osteoporosis) which can rule out certain exercise programs.

Be upbeat and make workouts enjoyable. Don't be afraid to add a little fun to the classes, such as wearing special hats or clothes on holidays. Acknowledge birthdays and show an interest in the client's lives.

If an instructor is enthusiastic, the enthusiasm is caught by the clients, and they *will* come back for more.

Visit new residents if you are working in a retirement facility. Inform them of what is available and encourage them to observe different fitness programs in session. Work with them to decide on a suitable program to fit their needs.

Program Description

The Village at Duxbury Fitness Program consists of muscle conditioning, cardiovascular endurance, flexibility, balance, improving posture, relaxation techniques and stress management.

The Fitness Center includes six (6) Keiser resistance machines (three lower body and three upper body), a treadmill, a Nustep (recumbent stair stepper and rower), free weights (barbells) and weight bench.

Programs in the Fitness Center are monitored, and each person has a record of what is accomplished each day. Each participant has their own folder to record progress. ACSM* guidelines are followed concerning repetitions and sets.

The Fitness Center is also the "Hub," or social center, of the community. People come and meet their friends to socialize here. Contests, games and parties are held on an ongoing basis to keep everyone coming back.

Class overview:

Exercise classes – A large meeting room is used for exercise classes in the morning. The advanced class meets from 8:15 - 9:00 a.m. The class begins with gentle stretches and progresses to a 15 minute low impact aerobic session. From there the class progresses to muscle conditioning using weights or dynabands and finishes with a stretching session.

Water aerobics – Water aerobics are offered every day. This is an energetic class and lasts about an hour. The class starts slowly and works up to a good cardiovascular workout, followed by conditioning and stretching. Resistance gloves and water woggles (noodles) are used in this class. An arthritis water class is also offered.

Chair exercise – This is a class for individuals who may have health issues and feel more comfortable sitting down. The class begins with about 10 minutes of seated aerobics and then proceeds to conditioning with weights or bands. Participants do get out of their chairs to do lower body work and balancing exercises.

Tai Chi and Yoga – These classes are offered in periodic sessions.

Any of the exercises can be modified for special health concerns.

Hours of operation:

The Fitness Center is open 24 hours a day, 7 days a week. The Center is supervised and classes are held Monday through Friday from 7:30 a.m. to 4:00 p.m.

Tips for successful programming:

- Instructors should be knowledgeable in their field, energetic and personable, personable, personable. It will make all the difference in the world to the program.

- The right music is important. Big Band step tapes are very popular. (See *Senior Fitness Videos & Books* in the *Resource* section of this manual.) Keep the aerobic music between 120 - 126 beats per minute. Class members also like marching and classical music. Finding the right music takes time, but it can make or break a class. Use meditation tapes for the cool-down and stretching segments.

Program Results

Eighty percent (80%) of the residents are involved in a fitness program. Their success has been dramatic. People have actually gotten rid of their canes. Very shy individuals have come out of their shells and have become involved in other activities as a result of their participation in the Fitness Center.

When people feel good, their attitude is good. With so many fit people, The Village at Duxbury is a very happy place.

Program Tip

- **Conduct contests**, hold seasonal events and motivational activities in order to keep participants challenged and coming back for more.

Sample contest: Collect pictures of residents when they were young. Post them on the fitness center bulletin board and have participants fill out contest forms as to "Who's Who?" Announce contest results and prizes at dinner.

*American College of Sports Medicine

The Village Fitness Calendar

Monday

| 7:30 am - 12:00 noon | **Resistance Training** Build muscular strength |

8:20 am — **Advanced Conditioning**
Aerobics, flexibility, strengthening, balance and coordination with weights

9:00 am — **General Conditioning**
Chair exercises for flexibility, strength, balance and coordination

10:00 am — **Aquatics**
Water aerobics and water walking, a great cardiorespiratory workout!

1:30 pm - 4:00 pm — **Resistance Training**
Build muscular strength

2:00 pm - 4:00 pm — **Enjoy the pool, do your own workout!**

Tuesday

7:30 am - 8:20 am — **Resistance Training**
Build muscular strength

8:20 am — **Advanced Conditioning**
Aerobics, flexibility, strengthening, balance and coordination with weights

9:00 am — **General Conditioning**
Chair exercises for flexibility, strength, balance and coordination

10:00 am — **Aquatics**
Water aerobics and water walking, a great cardiorespiratory workout!

11:00 am — **Resistive Training**
Reserved for Allerton House residents

1:30 pm — **Weight Conditioning**
Build muscular strength in a group setting using hand weights

2:00 pm - 3:00 pm — **The Village Walking Club**
Join Bonnie for a walk around the grounds at your own pace.

3:00 pm - 4:00 pm — **Resistive Training**
Build muscular strength

Wednesday

7:30 am - 12:00 noon — **Resistive Training**
Build muscular strength

8:20 am — **Advanced Conditioning**
Aerobics, flexibility, strengthening, balance and coordination with weights

SAMPLE HANDOUT

Wednesday (continued)

9:00 am — **General Conditioning**
Chair exercises for flexibility,
strength, balance and coordination

1:30 pm - 4:00 pm — **Resistive Training**
Build muscular strength

2:00 pm - 4:00 pm — **Enjoy the pool, do your own workout!**

Thursday

7:30 am - 8:20 am — **Resistive Training**
Build muscular strength

8:20 am — **Advanced Conditioning**
Aerobics, flexibility, strengthening,
balance and coordination with weights

9:00 am — **General Conditioning**
Chair exercises for flexibility,
strength, balance and coordination

10:00 am — **Aquatics**
Water aerobics and water walking,
a great cardiorespiratory workout!

11:00 am — **Resistive Training**
Reserved for Allerton House residents

1:00 pm — **Weight Conditioning**
Build muscular strength in a group
setting using hand weights

3:00 pm - 4:00 pm — **Resistance Training**
Build muscular strength

Friday

7:30 am - 12:00 noon — **Resistance Training**
Build muscular strength

8:20 am — **Advanced Conditioning**
Aerobics, flexibility, strengthening,
balance and coordination with weights

9:00 am — **General Conditioning**
Chair exercises for flexibility,
strength, balance and coordination –
using resistance bands

10:00 am — **Water Walking**
Join Bonnie Armstrong in her water walking
class…great aerobic workout! (1/2 hour of
water walking is equivalent to two hours of
land walking.)

1:30 pm - 4:00 pm — **Resistance Training**
Build muscular strength

2:00 pm - 4:00 pm — **Enjoy the pool, do your own workout!**

The Village at Duxbury

(Date Here)

Dear Dr. _____ :

_____ has requested participation in a **progressive cardiorespiratory endurance, flexibility and resistance training program.**

The resistance training program is modeled after the recently published research findings of the USDA's Human Nutrition Center on Exercise and Aging, at Tufts University in Boston (*The New England Journal of Medicine*, June 23, 1994). I have enclosed a copy of this article for your review. Due to the intensity of this program, I am requesting that you instruct me on any limitations your patient may have and on any restrictions you want to impose. The program is high intensity, progressive resistance training on major upper and lower body muscle groups, using Keiser air resistance equipment. Air resistance is safer than traditional weight stack equipment in that it eliminates shock loading to joints and provides consistent force throughout the range of motion. Initial training phase sessions are one hour long, 3 days per week for 10 weeks, and include cardiorespiratory warm-up, cool-down and stretching. For optimal strength gains, resistance is set at 80% of one repetition maximum (the maximal load that can be lifted fully one time only). After 10 weeks, training sessions are reduced to 2 days per week for maintenance of strength gains.

Research indicates that resistance training has little effect on blood pressure and heart rate. However, these will be monitored periodically. All programs are supervised and monitored carefully and will be terminated if any complications arise.

If you have any questions, Please call me at (617) 585-2334.

Yours truly,

Bonnie Armstrong

(Handout created using ACSM guidelines.)

Physician's Statement and Clearance Form

Information requested for: _____

Physician's Name: _____

Telephone Number: _____

Please check the statement that reflects your wishes.

_____ **I concur** with my patient's participation in a progressive cardiorespiratory endurance, resistance training and flexibility program.

_____ **I do not concur** with my patient's participation in this program.

_____ **I concur** with my patient's participation in a progressive cardiorespiratory endurance, resistance training and flexibility program, **with the following restrictions:**

_____

_____

_____

_____

_____

Signature _____ Date _____

Please return form to: Bonnie Armstrong
                         Fitness Coordinator
                         The Village at Duxbury
                         290 Kings Town Way
                         Duxbury, MA 02332

(Handout created using ACSM guidelines.)

NAME: _____

DATE: _____

	Setting ➡	Reps & Sets																
DATE																		
TREADMILL																		
LEG EXTENSION																		
LEG CURL																		
LEG PRESS																		
SEATED ROW																		
LAT PULLDOWN																		
CHEST PRESS																		
BICYCLE																		
NUSTEP																		

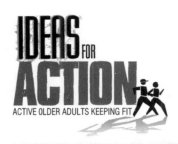

IDEAS FOR **ACTION**
ACTIVE OLDER ADULTS KEEPING FIT

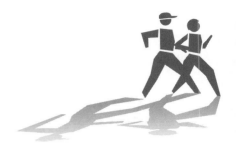

Vital Life Center – "It's Never Too Late to Start Feelin' Great"

Organization:	Vital Life Center
	3184 Collins Drive
	Merced, CA 95348
Phone:	(209) 723-2400
Fax:	(209) 723-3287
Contributor:	Gene Millen, President

Program Objective

- to provide a structured program geared toward the over 40 population

Materials/Equipment Needed

- Keiser compressed air strength training equipment

- Polar heart rate monitors

- equipment to assess aerobic capacity, strength, flexibility, body composition and cardiac risk evaluation

- functional fitness assessment using the resource, FUNCTIONAL FITNESS FOR ADULTS OVER 60 YEARS by Wayne Osness

Program Strategies

The target market of **Vital Life** is the over 40 population segment, most of whom are out of condition, are concerned about overdoing it and are reluctant to join a typical gym because they don't feel comfortable working out with the muscular young "jocks" and trim women in their 20's and 30's. Members are more interested in improving their health and vitality and shedding a few pounds than becoming a "hunk" or an athlete. They know that they should get more exercise for their health's sake, but don't have a clear understanding of what they should do or the discipline to be consistent. They need and appreciate the help of a structured program.

Program Description

Vital Life is unique in its approach of providing a coordinated program of personalized, monitored exercise and nutrition and stress management information *specifically designed for persons over 40.* This differs from the programs of health clubs which have traditionally catered to the younger market. These clubs usually offer their older adults a "senior" aerobics class, stretching class, aqua motion class or strength training class that meets two or three times per week at a specific time.

Vital Life takes a different approach. A complete structured program is offered on a daily basis. Older adults lead very busy and active lifestyles and appreciate the flexibility to exercise when it is convenient for them. Members may participate in the PROGRAM anytime the center is open – Monday through Friday from 5 AM to 8:30 PM and Saturday from 7 AM to 2 PM.

Each new member completes a HEALTH HISTORY which describes any physical limitations which need to be taken into consideration in developing an *individualized* EXERCISE PLAN for the member. The new members work at their own pace under the guidance of the EXERCISE SPECIALISTS who are always available to assist the members. The EXERCISE PLAN is updated frequently to insure that the member is challenged to continue improving their cardiovascular fitness, strength and flexibility.

Unique program concepts include the non-competitive atmosphere, warm "high touch" decor, high quality video/sound system and individualized attention to each member. The emphasis is on health, and members mention that one of the primary features that attracted them to **Vital Life** is the pleasant and non-competitive atmosphere.

Heart rates are monitored. Members are provided with a heart rate monitor and instructed on how to keep their heart rate in the "target zone." This minimizes the risk of over-exertion and assists in keeping the exercise activity at the optimum level. Blood pressure readings are taken before and after exercise and are kept in a computer data base for historical review and comparison.

Personal Health and Fitness Profile

This profile includes assessments of aerobic capacity, strength, flexibility, body composition and a cardiac risk evaluation. Functional fitness is also being implemented using the resource, FUNCTIONAL FITNESS FOR ADULTS OVER 60 YEARS by Wayne Osness. Periodic re-assessments are conducted to document the members' progress toward his/her goals and a graph is provided showing their improvements. Our monthly Newsletter features members who have shown significant improvements in their fitness, such as strength, blood pressure and other health markers.

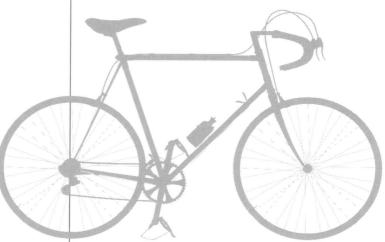

The program is fun, very informative and highly personalized. Humor plays an important role in the **Vital Life** program. A "family" atmosphere and spirit of camaraderie exists which makes people feel at home. Members are greeted by their first name as they arrive to exercise. Concurrently with exercise, video clips of musicals, comedy shows and health topics are shown to make the exercise enjoyable and the time "go faster." Social interaction and peer pressure are promoted to keep participants interested and motivated.

Strength Training is extremely important to this age group, as it will improve nearly every aspect of their lives – from carrying in the groceries, picking up the grandkids or going on that "dream" vacation. For each decade of life, beginning in their 30's, the average person loses five (5) pounds of lean muscle while gaining 15 pounds of body fat. Resistance training restores lost strength and muscle mass, speeds up the metabolism, accelerates body fat loss and provides a sense of well being and confidence.

Vital Life uses Keiser compressed air strength training equipment. The finger tip controls allow resistance to be set in one (1) pound increments.

Program Results

The **Vital Life** 50 plus membership has grown from zero to 280 persons in 3 1/2 years. In a recent membership survey, 99% indicated they would be "extremely likely" to recommend the center to a friend.

The Vital Life Social Program

The social program includes a variety of events.

- On a daily basis, members take time out to have lunch, coffee or a fat-free yogurt in our "Guilt Free Snackery."

- Every two weeks a "Bunko" game is held at **Vital Life**.

- Members participate in six to eight trips a year. A recent outing included chartering buses to San Francisco to see "PHANTOM OF THE OPERA." Two buses filled with **Vital Lifers** and friends traveled on a 100-mile round trip to see "STARS ON ICE." A two-day trip to Catalina Island attracted 40 people.

- On a periodic basis, a "Pasta Feed," featuring a low-fat menu, is provided at the **Center**.

Program Tip

The social events are a key element in the program. New friendships are made, and members get acquainted with other **Vital Life** members who participate in their exercise at other times of the day. A newcomer recently said, "You've got a lot going on here. You sure have some great trips."

VITAL LIFE CENTER
"It's Never Too Late To Start Feelin' Great"

EXERCISE LOG SHEET – Record minutes or repetitions

Week of _____ Name _____

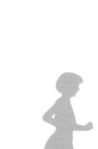

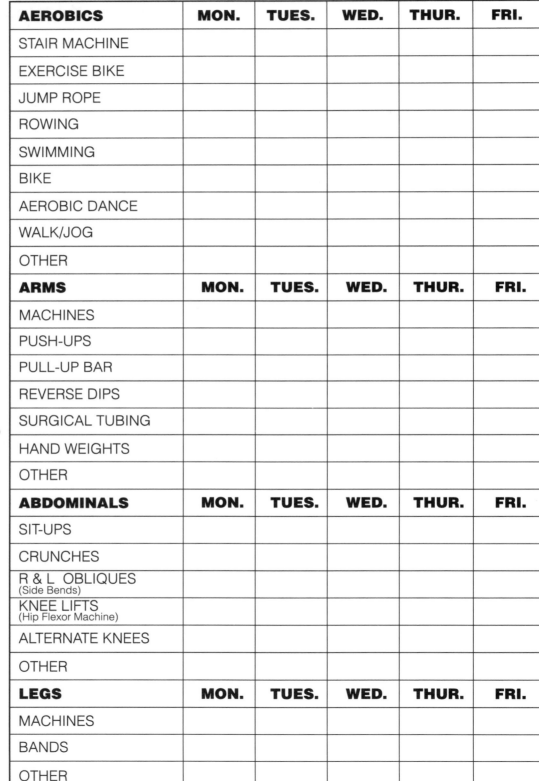

AEROBICS	MON.	TUES.	WED.	THUR.	FRI.
STAIR MACHINE					
EXERCISE BIKE					
JUMP ROPE					
ROWING					
SWIMMING					
BIKE					
AEROBIC DANCE					
WALK/JOG					
OTHER					
ARMS	**MON.**	**TUES.**	**WED.**	**THUR.**	**FRI.**
MACHINES					
PUSH-UPS					
PULL-UP BAR					
REVERSE DIPS					
SURGICAL TUBING					
HAND WEIGHTS					
OTHER					
ABDOMINALS	**MON.**	**TUES.**	**WED.**	**THUR.**	**FRI.**
SIT-UPS					
CRUNCHES					
R & L OBLIQUES (Side Bends)					
KNEE LIFTS (Hip Flexor Machine)					
ALTERNATE KNEES					
OTHER					
LEGS	**MON.**	**TUES.**	**WED.**	**THUR.**	**FRI.**
MACHINES					
BANDS					
OTHER					

VITAL LIFE CENTER

"It's Never Too Late To Start Feelin' Great"

EXERCISE LOG SHEET – Record minutes or repetitions

Week of _____ Name _____

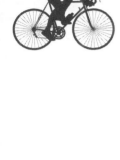

AEROBICS	MON.	TUES.	WED.	THUR.	FRI.

ARMS	MON.	TUES.	WED.	THUR.	FRI.

ABDOMINALS	MON.	TUES.	WED.	THUR.	FRI.

LEGS	MON.	TUES.	WED.	THUR.	FRI.

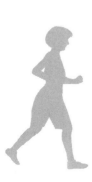

VITAL LIFE CENTER

"It's Never Too Late To Start Feelin' Great"

Personal Exercise Log

date	exercise mode	warm-up duration	exercise duration	cool-down duration	exercise HR	comments
Sun						
Mon						
Tue						
Wed						
Thu						
Fri						
Sat						

goals for next week:

Assessment Chart
VITAL LIFE CENTER

Name _____

Date	Weight	Body Composition	Aerobic Capacity	Flexibility	Strength

MUSCULAR FITNESS PROGRAM PLANNING FORM – VITAL LIFE CENTER

Name _____ Date _____ Class _____

Body Part	Exercise	Resistance	Repetitions	Sets

Comments: _____

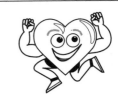

CARDIOVASCULAR FITNESS RECORD
(IS YOUR HEART GETTING STRONGER?)

Target Zone
(50%-75%)

Use the **F.I.T.** formula in order to improve the following:

FREQUENCY (How often)
INTENSITY (How hard)
TIME (How long)

DATE	RESTING PULSE RATE		DATE	RECOVERY RATE (5 Min.)
_____	_____		_____	_____
_____	_____		_____	_____
_____	_____		_____	_____
_____	_____		_____	_____
_____	_____		_____	_____
_____	_____		_____	_____
_____	_____		_____	_____
_____	_____		_____	_____
_____	_____		_____	_____
_____	_____		_____	_____

DATE	BLOOD PRESSURE		DATE	AEROBIC CAPACITY
_____	_____		_____	_____
_____	_____		_____	_____
_____	_____		_____	_____
_____	_____		_____	_____
_____	_____		_____	_____
_____	_____		_____	_____
_____	_____		_____	_____
_____	_____		_____	_____
_____	_____		_____	_____

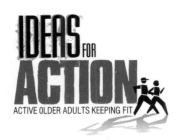

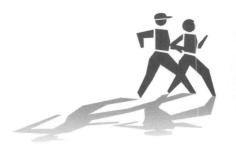

PROGRAM:

Walk Well

Organization: Hopkins Activity Center
33 14th Avenue North
Hopkins, MN 55343
Phone: (612) 939-1333
Fax: (612) 939-1342
Contributors: Debbie Vold/Susan Newville

Program Objectives

• to encourage participants to get active

• to motivate participants to be consistently active over a 20-week time span

Materials/Equipment Needed

• log cards

• biweekly tip sheets

• t-shirts and certificates for those who finish

Program Strategies

This program encourages and motivates participants to walk in hopes of helping them to develop a daily walking routine.

Program Description

"Walk Well" is an exercise incentive program which motivates participants to get active by following an imaginary route and tracking miles in a log book. The goal of participants is to complete 200 miles of walking in 20 weeks. Participants walk independently and record miles each day on a log card. Other activities can be converted to walking miles as per the conversion chart printed on the log card.

During this 20-week program, participants receive a biweekly incentive newsletter/tip sheet. Information about towns, attractions and parks is featured, as well as health/walking information.

Procedure

Hold a kick-off seminar to explain the program and distribute log cards. Review proper walking technique and explain the health benefits of a walking program.

At the end of 20 weeks, program participants turn in their log cards on the deadline date. All who finish the 200 miles within the 20-week time period, receive a certificate and a t-shirt.

Program Tips

- **Advertise** the "Walk Well" program through a variety of promotional means; i.e., flyers, newsletters, newspaper press releases.

- **Contact tourist information centers and chambers of commerce** for information about the area and cities the imaginary walk goes through.

- **Copy walking log sheet on cardstock** for durability.

- **Encourage the buddy system.** Have participants find a walking "buddy" for adherence and positive social interaction.

- **Hold an award ceremony** to present those who have completed the course their certificates and t-shirts. Invite the media.

WALK WELL

200 mile "imaginary" hike in 20 weeks. Enjoy the sights of Southeastern Minnesota as you walk, jog, bike, etc. your way to your 200 mile personal goal.

- *Newsletters*
- *Tracking map & log book*
- *T-shirt for finishers*

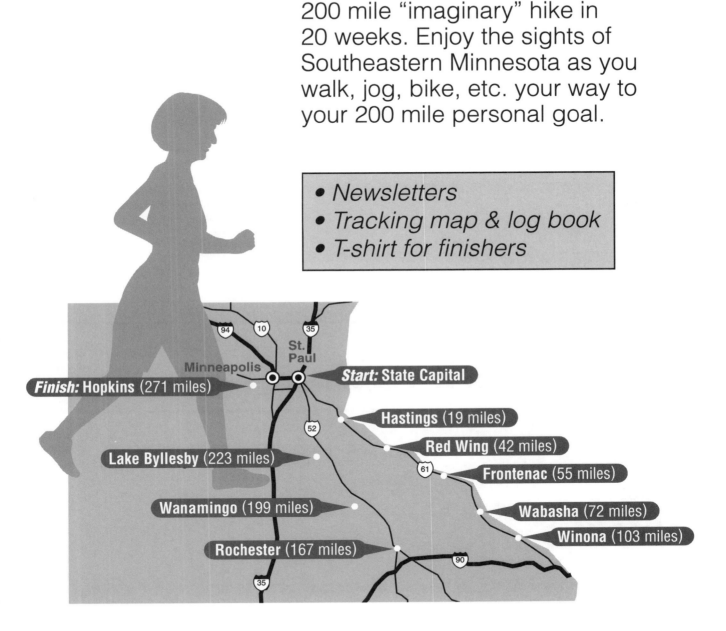

Minneapolis · St. Paul

Start: State Capital

Finish: Hopkins (271 miles)

Hastings (19 miles)

Red Wing (42 miles)

Lake Byllesby (223 miles)

Frontenac (55 miles)

Wanamingo (199 miles)

Wabasha (72 miles)

Winona (103 miles)

Rochester (167 miles)

TIP: When reproducing for handouts, copy pages 130 and 131 back to back.

"WALK WELL" Walking Program

WEEK											
MON											
TUES											
WED											
THURS											
FRI											
SAT											
SUN											
Weekly Total											
	Acc. Total										

"WALK WELL" Walking Program

WEEK											
MON											
TUES											
WED											
THURS											
FRI											
SAT											
SUN											
Weekly Total											
	Acc. Total										

SAMPLE HANDOUT

TIP: When reproducing for handouts, copy pages 130 and 131 back to back.

CONVERSION CHART

EQUIVALENTS TO ONE (1) MILE OF WALKING, ASSUME 15 MIN./MILE		
Activity	**# Min. or Miles = 1 Mile**	
Biking	.28 or	1.9
Nordic Track	.9.5 or	.6
Stairmaster	.11 or	.7
Rowing	.8.5 or	.6
Treadmill	.10 or	.7
Swimming	.7 or	.5
Jump-Rope	.10 or	1.0
Skating/In-line or Ice .	.24 or	1.6
Jogging/Running	.11 or	.7

WALKING PROGRAM
"WALK WELL"

**200 MILES
IN 20 WEEKS**

SPONSORED BY
(Your organization and
phone number here)

_____
NAME

CONVERSION CHART

EQUIVALENTS TO ONE (1) MILE OF WALKING, ASSUME 15 MIN./MILE		
Activity	**# Min. or Miles = 1 Mile**	
Biking	.28 or	1.9
Nordic Track	.9.5 or	.6
Stairmaster	.11 or	.7
Rowing	.8.5 or	.6
Treadmill	.10 or	.7
Swimming	.7 or	.5
Jump-Rope	.10 or	1.0
Skating/In-line or Ice .	.24 or	1.6
Jogging/Running	.11 or	.7

WALKING PROGRAM
"WALK WELL"

**200 MILES
IN 20 WEEKS**

SPONSORED BY
(Your organization and
phone number here)

_____
NAME

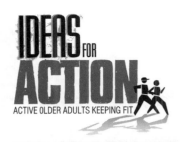

IDEAS FOR ACTION
ACTIVE OLDER ADULTS KEEPING FIT

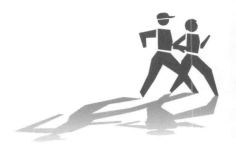

PROGRAM:

Water Walking

Organization: United States Water Fitness Association (USWFA)
P.O. Box 3279
Boynton Beach, FL 33424-3279
Phone: (561) 732-9908
Fax: (561) 732-0950
e-mail: uswfa@emi.net
Web-Site: www.emi.net/~uswfa/
Contributor: John R. Spannuth, President/CEO

Program Objective

- to promote water walking as a low impact, joint friendly exercise option

Materials/Equipment Needed

- pool
- water walking flyers (available from USWFA)

Program Description

Benefits of Exercising in the Water

- **Buoyancy:** This water property allows people to easily do exercises that are difficult on land. Ninety percent (90%) of the body is buoyant when in the water up to your neck, so you are not hitting the floor as hard as you would on land.

- **Resistance:** There is continual resistance to every move you make. The water offers 12%-14% more resistance than when you exercise on land. Resistance does not allow for sudden body movements.

- **Cooling Effect:** Water disperses heat more efficiently, so there is less chance of overheating. The water continuously cools the body. Exercise in the water is cooler and more comfortable than it is on land.

Water Walking

Water Walking is done in waist deep to chest deep water. If you do not have access to a pool at your facility, contact one or more of the following facilities or organizations.

- Health Clubs/Fitness Centers
- YMCA/YWCA/JCC
- Apartment Complexes/Condos
- Boy's & Girl's Clubs
- Colleges & Universities
- Mobile Home Parks
- Parks & Recreation Departments
- Physical Therapy/Sports Med. Centers

Inquire about the possibility of using their pool as a venue for Water Walking.

How to Start a Water Walking Program (Step by Step)

A. **Remember that the number of potential water walkers *far* exceeds the number of potential lap swimmers.** The USWFA estimates that approximately 8% of the people in the U.S. can swim laps. It is estimated that 98% of the population can walk in the water.

B. **Understand what water walking is and what it can do for participants.**

1. Read and study the water walking flyer.
2. Read a research paper: Example – *Comparison of Heart Rate Responses – Water Walking versus Treadmill Walking*, by Jim D. Whitley and Lori Schoene, *Physical Therapy Magazine*, Volume 67, Number 10, October 1987.

C. **Get approval to conduct a Water Walking program.**

D. **Decide what type of water walking program you will have.**

1. Formal

   a. Water walking seminar
   b. Water walking classes

      1. Beginner – Teach basic steps and provide a chance for people to water walk in a group.
      2. Intermediate/Advanced – Teach more advanced steps and get the heart rate up higher than in the beginner class.

   The KEY to having successful water walking classes is the instructor. The instructor must be a very enthusiastic and creative person who can keep people coming back...and get them to bring their friends!

2. Informal

   a. When will people be able to water walk – at times other than classes? Make sure the list of times is posted throughout the building and listed in program schedules, newsletters, etc.

3. Water Walking Club

   a. Activities

      1. Social events (covered dish, interesting speakers, holiday parties, etc.)
      2. Visit other swimming pools and water walk there.
      3. A simple, in-house newsletter, featuring success stories, training tips, programming ideas, etc.

E. **Promote the program's benefits.**

    1. In house (at your facility)

        a. Sell your staff on the program
        b. Post newspaper articles on bulletin boards
        c. Hand out water walking flyers (available from USWFA)
        d. Talk it up – sell people on the benefits
        e. Hold a free water walking seminar for your existing participants and other members – we suggest that you hold free seminars at least once each month

    2. Promote the program within the community.

        a. Letters to doctors, therapists, physical therapists, senior centers, etc.
        b. Article in local newspaper
        c. TV story (remember TV looks for success stories or unusual people)
        d. Free water walking seminar for the community several times a year
        e. Present a program to civic organizations such as Rotary, Kiwanis, etc. – these are usually 20 minute presentations at a lunch meeting – hand out water walking flyers

F. **Spend time in the halls and pool area talking to water walkers and potential water walkers.**

G. **Questions: Contact the USWFA at (561) 732-9908.**

How to Begin Water Walking

A. ***Never ever begin an exercise program or activity without the approval of your physician.***

B. **Don't over do it the first few times you Water Walk! Gradually work into Water Walking on a regular basis.**

C. **Each Water Walking session should consist of the following:**

    1. **WARM-UP –** Prepare your body for the exercise. Walk slowly stretching and taking it easy for about 3 to 5 minutes.
    2. **THE MAIN SET** of your exercise session. Build up to walking the amount of time you have allowed for your Water Walking session today. Progressively intensify your workout and speed your exercise up to the point that is proper for you.
    3. **COOL DOWN –** Use more gentle movements and give your body a chance to return gradually to its normal resting heart rate.

D. **We suggest that you Water Walk at *least* three (3) times a week.** If you only Water Walk three (3) times a week, try to do it on alternating days. Always allow one day of rest per week.

How to Water Walk

One of the great things about Water Walking is that you can be CREATIVE!
You can walk forward, backward and sidewards. You can use a variety of steps including regular steps, short quick steps, long steps, etc. You can move your arms in a variety of ways. Water Walking does not have to be boring! Listed below are ways to Water Walk.

A. **FORWARD**

    1. Normal steps

    2. Quick short steps

    3. Long steps (don't overdo it!)

    4. Step kicks

        a. alternate legs
        b. toe touches – touch your toe with your hand
        c. same leg kicks forward each time (change legs after each length)

    5. Knee touches – touch opposite knee with hand or elbow

    6. Circle steps – circle leg around to the side

    7. Move your arms in a variety of ways keeping your hands under the water

B. **BACKWARD**

    1. Normal steps

    2. Quick short steps

    3. Long steps (don't overdo it!)

    4. Kick back and step

    5. Move your arms in a variety of ways keeping your hands under the water

C. **SIDEWARDS**

    1. Legs do not cross

        a. Average size steps
        b. Raising the forward leg high, drop and then slide the back leg to it

    2. Cross over steps – cross one leg in front of the other and then cross that leg in back and step

    3. Side lunge

    4. Move your arms in a variety of ways keeping your hands under the water

Vary your workouts each day. Be creative!

Terms Used in Water Walking

A. **POSTURE (position of the body)**

   1. Don't slouch – but don't be too rigid

      a. Head upright (don't jut the jaw forward)
      b. Back straight
      c. Pull in the stomach and bottom
      d. Shoulders on a level plain – NOT tilted right or left – remember tight shoulders restrict breathing

B. **STRIDE (walk with long steps)**

   1. How to find your stride length

      a. Start in a standing position, lean forward at the ankles until you feel yourself falling forward. Then simply put your foot out to catch yourself. Look down. This is your stride length – no longer and no shorter. *Women's Sports and Fitness, May/June 1990*

C. **GAIT (manner of walking or stepping)**

D. **WATER WALKING SHOES**

   1. What are they? A soft, flexible shoe designed for walking in swimming pools, on boat decks, on the beach, etc.

   2. Why wear them?

      a. Comfort
      b. Eliminate wearing down of skin on the foot
      c. Protect feet
      d. Provide a non-skid base when walking on the pool deck, in the locker room and in the pool

   3. What kind of shoes to wear?

      a. Shoes designed for water fitness, boat decks, etc.
      b. Tennis shoes

Special Notes:

   *1. Water walkers should be **required** to wear water walking shoes in the pool!*

   2. Water walking shoes should only be worn from the person's locker to the pool and back – never outside the locker room or pool area! You never know what they might step on in the parking lot or other place, and then bring into your locker room or pool area on the bottoms of their feet!

E. **CIRCLE WALKING (discourage it!)**

   1. This would be like circle swimming, keeping your right arm close to the lane marker. We *completely discourage* circle walking because it reduces the amount of work being done by the participant. We encourage people to walk anywhere in the lane and "dodge" people if necessary.

Helpful Hints for Water Walking

By Paige Jackson, former USWFA National Technical Director

1. WALK ALL THE WAY THROUGH YOUR FOOT (toe and heel).

In the water, the tendency is to stay on your tiptoes. If you do stay on tiptoe, your legs don't get a full workload, only the calves are worked. *When walking forward* – step heel-to-toe, and when walking *backward* – step toe-to-heel. When jogging or running forward or backward – make sure to press heels down.

2. WALK (OR JOG) AN EQUAL NUMBER OF LAPS FORWARD AND BACKWARD.

To place equal emphasis on all muscles, you must travel both directions. Question: We don't walk backward on land, so why do we in the water? Answer: There is a continual resistance in the water, therefore, we are often using antagonistic muscle groups while we are walking a specific direction. To get a full range of motion and work all muscles evenly, we walk both directions.

3. WHILE WALKING TO THE SIDE (i.e., sidestep, grapevine, crabwalk) DON'T TURN AROUND AFTER EACH LENGTH. You must face the same direction (for example, the deep end) while walking both lengths or you won't work BOTH legs.

4. INCLUDE A WARM-UP AND COOL-DOWN IN YOUR WATER WALKING ROUTINE. In order to get the most benefit from your Water Walking workout and prevent injury or soreness, include a warm-up or stretch-out prior to heavy walking. If you are going to do an aerobic portion (jogging or using arms out of water), gradually increase your speed or arm movements. For example: take 2 minutes to stretch yourself out before you begin (on the deck or in the shallow water), then start with walking laps, building to marching, building to jogging. (Also build arm movements gradually.) When you see your time is almost up (last 5-7 minutes) begin slowing down gradually.

5. WAYS TO GET AN AEROBIC WORKOUT (INCREASE INTENSITY)

a. Jog or run
b. Use arms in water for muscular toning and endurance
c. Use arms out of water (cardiovascular endurance)
d. Lift knees higher
e. Lift arms higher – the higher your arms are, the harder your heart will work

6. BREATHE!

Don't forget to keep your breathing steady and take deep breaths (great for your cool down). On a high intensity workout, remember to blow your air out when you exert the most energy (i.e., when lifting knees high – blow air out). A great way to remember your breathing is to walk and talk with a friend.

7. THE MOST IMPORTANT HINT TO REMEMBER...HAVE FUN!

You have the freedom to be creative and make all your Water Walking laps different. It's a great way to stay fit and have a good time.

Safety

A. Major safety concerns:

1. Approval from physician before beginning program?

2. Don't overdo it!

3. When walking backward, be VERY careful! Alternate looking to the right and left over the shoulder for obstacles such as ladders, the end of the pool or other people.

Built In WARNING SIGNALS

Our body has certain warning signals that tell us when it is time to stop or slow down. We **strongly** recommend that you listen to your body! Some of the signals our body gives us that tells us it is time to stop or slow down are:

1. Abnormal heart action

2. Pain or pressure in the center of the chest, the arm or throat

3. Dizziness, lightheadedness, sudden incoordination, confusion, cold sweat, glassy stare, pallor, blueness or near fainting

4. Persistent rapid heart action even after you stop exercising

5. Flare up of arthritic condition

6. Nausea

7. Breathlessness

8. Shin splints

9. Side stitch

10. Charley horse or musclebound feeling

The above signals are not cause to panic, but rather for cooling down and stopping exercise, evaluating and readjusting your program. Consult your physician if symptoms persist.

Water Walking program option:

Play Water Walk Polo – similar to water polo, but played in a 4' deep pool, all ages and abilities can play

Equipment needed – two goals and a water polo ball

Program Note: See *U.S. Water Fitness Association* in the *Resource* section of this manual for information on materials available from the USWFA.

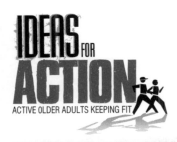

IDEAS FOR ACTION
ACTIVE OLDER ADULTS KEEPING FIT

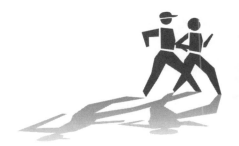

PROGRAM:

Young at Heart

Organization: Salem Athletic Club
16 Manor Parkway
Salem, NH 03079
Phone: (603) 893-8612
Fax: (603) 898-6211
Contributor: Kathy Kres, Young at Heart Director

Program Objective

• to promote health, fitness and friendship

Materials/Equipment Needed

• class specific – see individual class description for equipment needs

Program Description

Young at Heart is a program that is conducted within the Salem Athletic Club.

The program consists of approximately 250 Senior members who participate in social events, aerobics and water classes, as well as utilize the club's exercise equipment.

Emphasis is evenly balanced between the social and fitness aspect.

Procedures and Teaching Strategies

Essential Ingredients for a SENIOR Exercise Class

Experienced and Knowledgeable Instructors

• certification/training in exercise, education, fitness, health related fields

• enjoyment and understanding of older adults and their concerns

• familiarity with medical conditions commonly found with older adults – arthritis, stroke, cardiac disease, osteoporosis, limb amputation, neurologic diseases (dementia), depression, sight and hearing loss

Safety

- medical clearance for participants
- safe physical environment for exercise – lighting, stairs, parking, phone access
- safe learning environment – low emotional risk, acceptance of all
- ability to recognize exercise stress signals of participants
- good judgment and appropriate action in response to medical emergencies

LOVE

- esteem for all people of all ages, open-mindedness
- sincerity in the holistic well-being of participants – actions and words
- social support and gatherings – presence, courtesy, tactfulness, holidays
- sensitivity to atmosphere and mood of the moment

Fun

- sense of humor is a must – look on the bright side of life
- make it enjoyable – LAUGH – be ridiculous! (at least once in a while)
- share personal experiences, joke, tell stories, pass out cartoons, use theatrics (hats, costumes), celebrate "special days," plan for holidays

Relevancy

- educate participants about specific benefits to be gained from activities, e.g. strengthening, mobility, independence, nutrition, health, wellness
- use handouts, newspaper articles, health letters, and other educational tools to keep people informed and interested in their health

Variety of Activities

- use a core of familiar activities that exercise the entire body
- introduce new exercises and ideas gradually – don't make them too easy or too difficult

Motivation

- enthusiasm – be the most positive and enthusiastic person you know!
- make it easy to participate and to succeed – provide mental stimulation and challenge

Maturation

- levels of maturity differ from one area to another – intellectual, physical, emotional, social
- experiences (work, family, career) affect us all uniquely over the years – consider this when instructing, educating and relating

Encouragement

- recognize humanness – "It's not easy!" "What an effort!" "Try it again!"
- remind people of the next class meeting time
- suggest exercising between classes

Feedback

- correct performance of exercises
- offer support and recognition for effort and improvement
- listen carefully to the conversations your participants share and respond accordingly (in reference to neurologic diseases)

Additional Considerations

- address participants by name

- make eye contact with each individual in your class – smile

- vary tone of voice, pitch, enthusiasm and rhythm

- keep directions simple

- use vocabulary and imagery that describes the exercise movement

- choose appropriate music that fits your class participants' age and activity level

- end the class in a positive manner

Safety Considerations for Elder Exercise – Instructor Information

Medical Consent: Prior to starting any exercise program, it is a necessary requirement for a class participant to get a physician's consent or medical waiver to participate (see page 149). This is critical for the participant *and* for you as an instructor.

Adverse Responses to Exercise: Commonly accepted responses to exercise include increased rate of breathing, a feeling of bodily warmth and muscle fatigue. These are normal, even for elder exercisers. When working with elders, special attention must be paid to observing outward signs of physical distress and fatigue that could possibly lead to a more dangerous situation. As an instructor, you need to be able to identify exercise stress signs, particularly for elders who may not verbalize well or are unable to speak at all. The following is a list of responses:

- unusual fatigue

- throbbing head

- tightness or pain in the chest, arms, back, throat or jaw

- abnormal heart response – very fast, fluttering/palpitations

- severe breathlessness

- lightheadedness, sudden confusion, dizziness

- loss of muscle control or balance, shakiness, trembling

- cold sweat

- sudden weakness or numbness in the face, arm or leg

- nausea, queasiness, vomiting

If any participant exhibits any of these responses, have them stop exercising immediately and alert medical personnel as the situation necessitates. Maintain your composure, stay with the person who is in distress, and find someone to help with your class if available. Document the event by completing a written incident report (see pages 150 and 151).

Emergencies: Plan procedures that will be followed in case of an emergency. Know where the nearest telephone is and the emergency number. Do not hesitate to call for medical assistance if you think that you need it...just do it. Keep your participants' medical consent forms nearby in case you need to give any of their medical information to emergency personnel.

Arthritis: Participants with arthritis should not exercise with weights when joints are red, inflamed, swollen and hot. A limited number of repetitions or simple range of motion for flexibility and mobility is adequate.

Chairs and Wheelchairs: Use sturdy chairs for exercise. Have some chairs with arms and some without arms. Check to see that the chairs do not slide if class is held in a room with a linoleum floor. Set wheelchair brakes so that they do not roll during seated as well as standing exercise.

Monitoring Participants' Exercise Response: The Borg Scale of Perceived Exertion is one way to monitor how hard participants are exercising (see chart below). Explain the scale to them prior to starting classes and during classes. Periodically ask them how hard they feel that they are working.

Rate of Perceived Exertion Scale

6	
7	Very, very light
8	
9	Very light
10	
11	Fairly light
12	
13	Somewhat hard
14	
15	Hard
16	
17	Very hard
18	
19	Very, very hard
20	

Perceived exertion is a method used to monitor exercise intensity. Select a rating that corresponds to your subjective perception of how hard you are exercising when training within your target heart rate zone. As you exercise, you will become familiar with the amount of exertion required to raise your heart rate to your target level by using the Rate of Perceived Exertion Scale.

Participants working at a 10 to 14 exertion level are working at an acceptable range. Level 15 and above is too high. Participants need to be told to slow down and take it easier.

Offer alternatives for people if they are fatigued. Suggest that they stop and rest. When people have been standing and exercising, suggest that they sit down and finish the exercises sitting, if they have the energy to do that.

Exercise Equipment: Caution class participants about placement of exercise equipment. Put dumbbells, stretch ropes and ankle weights under chairs when not being used. If people use canes or walkers, find a safe, yet accessible, place for them.

The Pros of Strength Training and the Elder Exerciser

Just why should Seniors strength train? And what specifically should you tell them about the benefits of working out with weights? Wayne L. Westcott, Ph.D., fitness research director at the South Short YMCA (Quincy, MA), summarizes the reasons why adults – of any age – should strength train:

- *It prevents muscle loss and increases muscle mass.* Adults lose an average of six pounds of muscle per decade. Resistance training preserves muscle mass and strength.

- *It increases the body's metabolic rate.* During each decade, the average adult has a 2 to 5 percent reduction in metabolic rate. Adding three pounds of muscle, however, can increase metabolic rate by 7 percent.

- *It increases bone-mineral density.* Studies show that older people who strength train can increase bone density in the spine and upper femur.

- *It improves glucose metabolism.* Researchers found that glucose uptake increases by 23 percent after just four months of strength training.

- *It reduces body fat.* In a recent study, researchers found that people who strength trained for three months lost four pounds of fat, even though they upped their daily calorie intake by 15 percent.

- *It increases gastrointestinal transmit time.* This can reduce the risk of colon cancer.

- *It lowers resting blood pressure.* And when done in tandem with aerobic exercise, it can improve blood-pressure readings even more.

- *It can improve blood lipid levels.*

- *It can reduce low-back pain.* People who experience low-back pain report less pain after 10 weeks of strength-training exercises that target the lower spine.

- *It can reduce the pain of arthritis.*

Description of Classes Offered in the Young at Heart Program

Above the Belt

Reason offered: to increase upper body functional strength and range of motion in all major upper body muscles and also to promote muscle balance

Classes per week: two (2)

Class description: "Above the Belt" consists of a series of exercises designed to increase functional strength in the arms, shoulders, chest and upper back. Hand-held weights (1 - 5 pounds) and resistance tubing are used in this class.

Below the Belt

Reason offered: to increase tone and strength in legs, hips, back, abdominals and glutials

Classes per week: three (3)

Class description: "Below the Belt" consists of a series of exercises designed to strengthen the lower part of the body as well as to tone and increase range of motion.

Stretch & Flex

Reason offered: to help increase range of motion and flexibility

Classes per week: three (3)

Class description: "Stretch & Flex" consists of a warm-up of the body to raise core temperature in order to improve range of motion and flexibility. In a dimly lit room with a background of soft music, participants are encouraged through slow-paced stretches to increase flexibility while using simple breathing techniques.

Water Walking

Reason offered: to increase exercise options for seniors, persons with physical limitations and those in rehabilitation

Classes per week: organized classes two (2) times a week – the pool is available before and after other classes for water walking

Class description: warm-up followed by walking in waist- or chest-deep water to music, followed by stretching

Water Walking is used by members in addition to regularly offered classes to further increase cardiovascular endurance. It is also used by those who are physically uncomfortable with gym exercises. Water Walking is a great place to start developing strength, endurance and balance.

Recommended as a beginner level class.

Walking Club

Reason offered: to increase cardiovascular endurance and offer an alternative to Gym Aerobics

Classes per week: five (5)

Program description: The "Walking Club" consists of a slow walk for about five (5) minutes with leg stretches. Then the pace is picked up to a comfortable walking/working level for the individual walker. Walk totals 2 1/2 miles at 12 - 15 minutes per mile.

Young-at-Heart Gym Exercise with Toning

Reason offered: to introduce toning/muscle strengthening to seniors

Classes per week: three (3)

Class description: This class incorporates toning exercises done with light hand weights, resistance bands, and tubing for upper and lower body toning. Floor exercises tone and strengthen abdominal muscles.

Young-at-Heart Water Exercise

Reason offered: to offer water exercises for seniors

Classes per week: five (5)

Class description: "Water Exercise" class complements gym exercise by providing the addition of range-of-motion exercises to help alleviate joint stiffness, arthritis, etc.

Supportive environment of the water allows those members with balance problems, joint injuries, back problems and other physical limitations to participate.

Young-at-Heart Gym Exercise

Reason offered: to offer specialty low-impact classes for seniors

Classes per week: five (5)

Class description: consists of low and non-impact aerobics with a warm-up/aerobic segment/cool down and stretch done to "Golden Oldies" music – incorporates a sense of humor into the class.

Young-at-Heart Lunch Bunch

Reason offered: to increase cohesiveness of group and have fun!

How often program runs: two (2) to three (3) times monthly

Program description: This group goes to lunch at area restaurants or at the Club's Cafe. Special trips may include dinner theaters, mystery lunches, and foliage cruises.

This is a great retention tool. The Seniors work together to carpool and provide rides for those who can't drive, so that all who wish to can participate. This social group becomes part of our members' lives and allows them to branch out into activities they might not do individually.

Young-at-Heart Coffee Social

Reason offered: to promote cohesiveness/retention of group

Meetings per week: five (5)

Program description: Pre-exercise social half hour where members meet with/visit with/encourage each other. This allows the group to celebrate birthdays, special events and achievements. Instructors serve coffee, muffins and bagels and have one-on-one contact with the members.

We feel this daily half hour is probably the key to the success of our program as a whole. The effortless assimilation of new enrollees and the long term social bonds that are formed encourage more frequent and longer term participation by members. The increased attendance helps them see better results from the exercise program. Psychologically, the friendship and chance to "get out of the house" is invaluable to many of our members who are widowed and/or live alone. It also gives the instructors an opportunity to get feedback on new or old programs and adjust their planning accordingly.

Arthritis Foundation Aquatic Program

Reason offered: to provide a program for persons with Arthritis to exercise, meet others who also have Arthritis and have fun

Classes per week: three (3)

Program description: Program participants are led by trained instructors through a series of specially designed exercises which, with the aid of the water's buoyancy and resistance, can help improve joint flexibility. The warm water and gentle movements also help to relieve pain and stiffness.

Program Results

Program members report weight loss, renewed energy levels, improved physical and mental health and valuable new friendships.

Program Tips

- Program emphasis should be **50% on physical activity and 50% social interaction.**

- **Hold an open house** to showcase the Seniors program. Be sure to serve refreshments.

- **Offer to give a luncheon talk** on fitness to a community service organization, i.e., Kiwanis, Lions, etc. to promote your program.

The "Trick" With Any Exercise Program Is To STICK WITH IT!!!

1. TAKE IT EASY…
While you're getting into shape. Don't expect to overcome years of inactivity in a few days. Mix exercise with every day activities whenever possible.

2. TWO'S COMPANY…
Have a friend or family member join you during your exercise breaks.

3. KEEP IN MIND…
The good things that exercise does for your heart, your looks and your spirit. Fitness is fun when you keep these goals in sight.

4. TAKE A SNAPSHOT…
of yourself (full-length, side view) to record your progress. On the back jot down your weight and resting pulse rate. "Measure up" every month – you'll notice the difference.

Other Ingredients In The Prescription For A Healthy Heart:

1. EAT RIGHT…
Have three (3) balanced meals. Watch calories, the kind and amount of fat. Cut down on rich treats and late night snacking.

2. LEARN TO RELAX…
A change of pace is a big help. Try breathing deeply and slowly while lying down.

3. GET ENOUGH REST…
Plenty of sleep every night gives you "go-power" for an active day.

4. AVOID WORRY AND STRESS…
Some stress is part of everyone's life. Exercise relieves excess tension. (Note: Smoking, alcohol and other drugs are not effective ways to relieve stress.)

Waiver

This program is under the direction of

_____ .

I understand that the benefits from participating in this group include learning more about the benefits of an active lifestyle and meeting my own goals.

I state that I am free from heart disease and other medical conditions, or that I have written permission from my doctor to participate in this program.

I release the sponsoring organization(s) and personnel from any responsibility or liability for any injury or health consequences that may result from my participation in this program.

My signature indicates that I have full knowledge of the purpose of the program, the benefits I may expect, and the risks involved. I agree to participate on this basis.

_____ _____

(signature)   (date)

_____ _____

(address)   (telephone #)

TIP: When reproducing, copy pages 150 and 151 back to back.

ACCIDENT CHECK LIST

Name (Last)   First   M.I.   Date (Month/Year)

_____   _____

Time (Hour:Minutes)   Location   Male   Female   Age

_____   _____   (Circle One)   _____

SUSPECTED CAUSE OF INJURY OR ILLNESS

☐ Non-Injury Ailment   ☐ Blunt Trauma   ☐ Hyper Extension   ☐ Hyper Flexion

☐ Rotation   ☐ Fall   ☐ Exposure   _____Other

SIGNS AND SYMPTOMS

☐ Contusion   ☐ Abrasion   ☐ Laceration   ☐ Bleeding

☐ Burn   ☐ Head Injury   ☐ Convulsions   ☐ Vomiting/ Nausea

☐ Visual Disturbances ☐ Hearing Disturbances ☐ Strain   ☐ Sprain

☐ Dislocation   ☐ Fracture   ☐ Crushed   ☐ Swelling

☐ Loss of Function   ☐ Discoloration   ☐ Pain   ☐ Numbness

☐ Heart Involvement   ☐ Lung Involvement   ☐ Abdominal Involvement   ☐ Shock

Other _____

Complaining of _____

SITE OF INJURY AND/OR ILLNESS

☐ None   ☐ Front   ☐ Back   ☐ Side

☐ Head/Face   ☐ Knee   ☐ Multiple   ☐ Eye(s)

☐ Mouth   ☐ Nose   ☐ Ear(s)   ☐ Lower Leg

☐ Bodywide   ☐ Neck   ☐ Shoulder   ☐ Chest

☐ Abdomen   ☐ Ankle   ☐ Pelvic Area   ☐ Upper Arm

☐ Elbow   ☐ Lower Arm   ☐ Foot   ☐ Wrist

☐ Hand   ☐ Fingers   ☐ Upper Leg   ☐ Toe(s)

TIP: When reproducing, copy pages 150 and 151 back to back.

ACCIDENT CHECK LIST *Continued*

PROCEDURES USED

☐ Airway Cleared or Opened   ☐ Artificial Ventilation   ☐ Oxygen Administered

☐ C.P.R.   ☐ Bleeding Control   ☐ Dressing   ☐ Bandaged   ☐ Compression

☐ Immobilization   ☐ Elevation   ☐ Administration of_____

☐ Stress Testing   ☐ Visual Testing   ☐ Motion Testing   ☐ Referred to:

_____

VITAL SIGNS

BLOOD PRESSURE   PULSE   RESP.

_____ / _____   _____   _____

PUPILS: ☐ Equal   ☐ Unequal   ☐ Dilated   ☐ Light Reactive
            ☐ Constricted   ☐ Fixed

MENTAL STATE: ☐ Conscious   ☐ Disoriented   ☐ Unconscious

RESPONSE TO PAIN: ☐ Yes   ☐ No

SKIN CONDITION: ☐ Normal   ☐ Cyanotic   ☐ Pale/Ashen   ☐ Flushed
                    ☐ Hot/Dry   ☐ Sweating

SPEECH: ☐ Normal   ☐ Slurred   ☐ Incoherent

PATIENT HISTORY:_____

_____

_____
Administrator's Signature

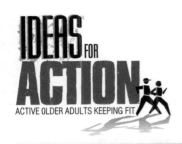

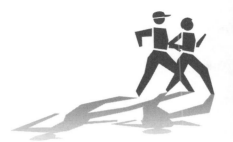

Part II

Resources

The following is a list of resources related to and supporting senior fitness. Resources listed are by no means all of the resources available.

Inclusion in this section of IDEAS FOR ACTION does not constitute an endorsement by the Sporting Goods Manufacturers Association.

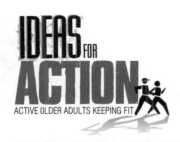

IDEAS FOR ACTION
ACTIVE OLDER ADULTS KEEPING FIT

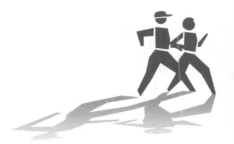

Aerobics and Fitness Association of America (AFAA)

Aerobics and Fitness Association of America
15250 Ventura Blvd., Suite 200
Sherman Oaks, CA 91403-3297

Phone: (818) 905-0040 or (800) 225-2322
Fax: (818) 990-5468
Web-Site: www.afaa.com

Organization Objective

- to provide educational workshops and certifications for fitness instructors

Program Description

Fitness instructors can choose from a variety of special population workshops as well as the following training and certifications:

- AFP Fitness Practitioner
- Practical Teaching Skills
- Step Teaching Skills
- Personal Trainer/Fitness Counselor
- Weight Training
- Emergency Response
- Primary Aerobic Instructor
- Step Certification

AFAA's fitness library includes many valuable educational resources for the professional fitness instructor. Home study courses include:

- Senior Fitness
- Aquatic Fitness
- Nutrition Fundamentals
- Exercise & Obesity
- plus many more

Additional AFAA resources include:

- Fitness Gets Personal cards – Written by experts in the field, these information cards provide facts and guidelines on a variety of exercise, nutrition, lifestyle and health/safety topics.

- 1-800-YOUR-BODY – A toll-free fitness hotline offering three free minutes of advice and optional one-on-one expert counseling.

- Fitness Triage – Fitness and allied health professionals participate in the nation's first integrated health and fitness advice and referral system.

- Emergency Response Certification – This workshop (open to everyone) is for anyone who wants to be able to identify and respond to emergency illnesses and injuries.

For more information, contact AFAA at the address above.

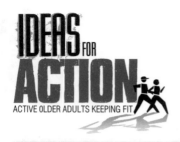

IDEAS FOR ACTION
ACTIVE OLDER ADULTS KEEPING FIT

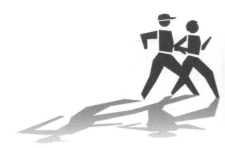

RESOURCE:

Amateur Athletic Union – Presidential Sports Award

Amateur Athletic Union (AAU)
Walt Disney Resorts
P.O. Box 10000
Lake Buena Vista, FL 32830-1000

Phone: (407) 363-6170
Fax: (407) 934-7242
Web-Site: aausports.org

Organization Description

The AAU is a non-profit organization of 300,000 members nationwide and is open to men and women interested in organizing or promoting amateur sports.

The AAU administers the Presidential Sports Award Program, which was developed by the President's Council on Physical Fitness and Sports (PCPFS) in 1972 in conjunction with national sports organizations and associations. Its purpose is to motivate all Americans to become more physically active throughout life and emphasizes regular fitness activity rather than outstanding performance.

Program Description

The President's Council on Physical Fitness and Sports is encouraging all Americans to be physically fit by offering its Presidential Sports Award (PSA) to individuals who exercise on a consistent, long-term basis.

Participants have four months to fulfill the requirements established for each category. There are **68 categories** to choose from.

Individuals who earn an award receive a personalized certificate of achievement from the President, a letter of congratulations from the Council, an impressive embroidered emblem signifying the sport in which the award was earned, a sports bag tag, and a shoe pocket to hold ID information while exercising.

Program brochures and additional category information for both group programs and individual ones may be obtained free of charge by sending a stamped, self-addressed envelope to:

Presidential Sports Award
AAU
Walt Disney Resorts
P.O. Box 10000
Lake Buena Vista, FL 32830-1000

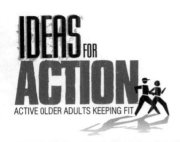

IDEAS FOR ACTION
ACTIVE OLDER ADULTS KEEPING FIT

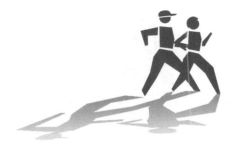

RESOURCE:

American Council on Exercise (ACE)

American Council on Exercise
5820 Oberlin Drive
San Diego, CA 92121

Phone: (800) 825-3636
Fax: (619) 535-1778
Web-Site: www.acefitness.org

Organization Description

The non-profit American Council on Exercise (ACE) is committed to promoting active, healthy lifestyles and their positive effects on the mind, body and spirit. ACE pledges to enable all segments of society to enjoy the benefits of physical activity and protect the public against unsafe and ineffective fitness products and instruction. ACE accomplishes its mission by setting certification and education standards for fitness instructors and through ongoing public education about the importance of exercise.

Educational materials for the senior market include:

ACE Fit Facts: one page informational sheets on more than 70 health and fitness topics including:

• Arthritis & Exercise
• Heart Disease & Exercise
• Osteoporosis Prevention

• Seniors & Fitness
• Starting an Exercise Program
• Making Time for Exercise

Callers can get up to three *ACE Fit Facts* free. Complete sets can be purchased.

Exercise for Older Adults – ACE's Guide for Fitness Professionals : This brand-new resource guide is an essential tool in the design of exercise programs for older clients. It includes information on the physiology of aging, health challenges faced by older adults, and exercise techniques and programming.

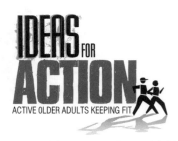

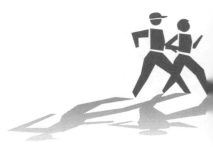

American Senior Fitness Association (SFA)

American Senior Fitness Association (SFA)
P.O. Box 2575
New Smyrna Beach, FL 32170
Phone: (800) 243-1478 or (904) 423-6634
Fax: (904) 427-0613

Organization Description

The American Senior Fitness Association was founded in 1992 with the primary goal of providing quality educational programs and recognized professional certification for fitness professionals who serve older adult populations. SFA programs were designed to enhance the skills of exercise professionals who hold academic degrees and/or general population exercise certification, as well as to provide senior-specific training for capable, motivated persons currently conducting senior fitness programs with little formal training. SFA operates under the technical guidance of a multi-disciplinary National Advisory Board which includes nationally recognized fitness experts. All of SFA's programs have been extensively researched, peer reviewed and thoroughly field tested to give fitness professionals the knowledge and confidence they need to successfully serve this rewarding market with the highest quality fitness programming available. SFA programs have been accepted for continuing education by many other associations.

SFA is increasingly becoming involved in membership support services and networking, as well as becoming a resource "clearinghouse" for older adult fitness information.

To meet the need for senior specific fitness education and practical training, SFA has developed three distinct learning tracks.

- Senior Fitness Instructor – designed for those who lead active, independent-living older adults in group exercise classes

- Senior Personal Trainer – designed for those who prefer to work one-on-one or in smaller groups focusing on personalized strength, aerobic and functional fitness

- Long Term Care Fitness Leader – designed for those who work with frail elderly persons in settings such as nursing homes, adult day care and adult congregate living facilities

For more information contact SFA at (800) 243-1478 or (904) 423-6634.

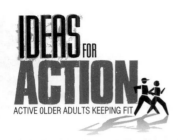

ACTIVE OLDER ADULTS KEEPING FIT

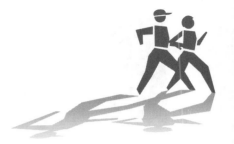

Arthritis Foundation YMCA Aquatic Program (AFYAP/PLUS)

Arthritis Foundation
1330 W. Peachtree Street
Atlanta, GA 30309
Phone: (800) 283-7800
Fax: (404) 872-0457
Web-Site: www.arthritis.org

Program Description

The Arthritis Foundation and the YMCA of the USA developed these aquatic programs as a joint venture. Instructor training is available through your local chapter of the Arthritis Foundation. For a complete listing of services available in your area, contact your local chapter of the Arthritis Foundation. Call (800) 283-7800 for chapter information.

An overview of AFYAP exercises:

AFYAP exercises are geared toward those parts of the body commonly affected by arthritis. They are designed to increase range-of-joint motion and muscular strength. Multiple exercises are provided for the neck, trunk, shoulders, elbows, wrists and fingers, chest, hips and knees, and ankles and toes, as well as for the lower-extremity and abdominal areas and walking.

An overview of AFYAP PLUS exercises:

Although AFYAP PLUS includes a longer endurance component than the basic AFYAP program, it is not a high-intensity aerobic conditioning program. The activities should be performed at a low to moderate intensity in order to improve muscular strength and endurance with a minimum risk of injury. As in the basic AFYAP, it is important to use good body posture and proper body mechanics while doing the AFYAP PLUS activities.

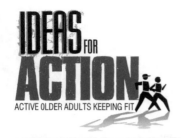

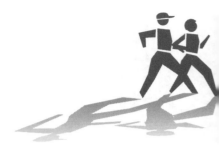

RESOURCE:

Associations & Organizations Offering Senior Sports Opportunities

The Adventure Cycling Association
P.O. Box 8308
Missoula, MT 59807
Phone: (406) 721-1776
Fax: (406) 721-8754
e-mail: acabike@aol.com
Web-Site: www.adv-cycling.org

The Amateur Athletic Union (AAU)
Walt Disney Resorts
P.O. Box 10000
Lake Buena Vista, FL 32830-1000
Phone: (407) 363-6170
Fax: (407) 934-7242
e-mail: jeanann@aausports.org
Web-Site: aausports.org

Amateur Softball Association (ASA)
2801 NE 50th Street
Oklahoma City, OK 73111
Phone: (405) 424-5266
Fax: (405) 424-3855
Web-Site: www.softball.org

Amateur Speedskating Union of the U.S.
1033 Shady Lane
Glen Ellyn, IL 60137-4822
Phone: (630) 790-3230
Fax: (630) 790-3235

American Alpine Club (AAC)
710 10th Street
Golden, CO 80401
Phone: (303) 384-0110
Fax: (303) 384-0111
Web-Site: www.americanalpineclub.org

American Platform Tennis Association
P.O. Box 43336
Upper Montclair, NJ 07043
Phone: (973) 744-1190
Fax: (973) 783-4407
Web-Site: www.platformtennis.org

American Running and Fitness Association (ARFA)
4405 East West Highway, Suite 405
Bethesda, MD 20814
Phone: (301) 913-9520
Fax: (301) 913-9517
e-mail: arfarun@aol.com
Web-Site: www.arfa.org

American Walking Association
P.O. Box 4
Paonia, CO 81428-0004
Phone: (970) 527-4557
Fax: (970) 527-4607

American Water Ski Association
799 Overlook Drive
Winterhaven, FL 33884
Phone: (800) 533-2972
Fax: (941) 325-8259
e-mail: usawaterski@worldnet.att.net
Web-Site: usawaterski.org

Bowling Inc.
5301 South 76 Street
Greendale, WI 53129
Phone: (414) 421-6400
Fax: (414) 421-1650

Ice Skating Institute
355 West Dundee Road
Buffalo Grove, IL 60089
Phone: (847) 808-7528
Fax: (847) 808-8329
e-mail: skateisi@aol.com
Web-Site: www.skateisi.com

**International In-Line Skating
  Association**
3720 Farragut Avenue, Suite 400
Kensington, MD 20895
Phone: (301) 942-9770
Fax: (301) 942-9771
e-mail: iisahq@erols.com
Web-Site: www.iisa.org

International Jugglers Association
P.O. Box 218
Montague, MA 01351
Phone: (413) 367-2401
Fax: (413) 367-0259
e-mail: ijugglersa@aol.com
Web-Site: www.juggle.org

**International Senior Softball
  Association**
9401 East Street
Manasas, VA 20110
Phone: (703) 368-1188
Fax: (703) 368-3411

League of American Bicyclists
1612 K Street NW, Suite 401
Washington, DC 20006
Phone: (202) 822-1333
Fax: (202) 822-1334
e-mail: bikeleague@aol.com
Web-Site: www.bikeleague.org

**Men's Senior Baseball League
  (MSBL)**
1 Huntington Quadrangle, Suite 3N07
Melville, NY 11747
Phone: (516) 753-6725
Fax: (516) 753-4031
e-mail: msblnational@msbl.com
Web-Site: www.msbl.com

**National Congress of State Games
  & Member States (NCSG)**
401 North 31 Street
Billings, MT 59101
Phone: (406) 254-7426
Fax: (406) 254-7439
e-mail: Tom@stategames.org
Web-Site: www.stategames.org

**National Horseshoe Pitchers
  Association (NHPA)**
3085 76th Street
Franksville, WI 53126
Phone and Fax: (414) 835-9108
Web-Site: www.geocities.com/~NHPA

National Senior Games Association
445 North Boulevard, Suite 2001
Baton Rouge, LA 70802
Phone: (504) 379-7337
Fax: (504) 379-7343

**National Senior Sports Association -
  Golf Division**
83 Princeton Avenue
Hopewell, NJ 08525
Phone: (800) 282-6772
Fax: (609) 466-9366
Web-Site: www.amgolftour.com

North American Senior Circuit Softball (NASCS)
1204 West 46 Street
Richmond, VA 23225
Phone: (804) 231-4254 or (810) 791-2632
Fax: (804) 232-4539

North American Telemark Organization
Box 44
Waitsfield, VT 05673
Phone: (800) 835-3404

Professional Bowlers Association of America
1720 Merriman Road
Akron, OH 44334
Phone: (330) 836-5568
Fax: (330) 836-2107
Web-Site: www.pbatour.com

Rails to Trails Conservancy
1100 17th Street NW, 10th Floor
Washington, DC 20036
Phone: (202) 331-9696
Fax: (202) 331-9680
e-mail: rtrails@transact.org
Web-Site: www.railtrails.org

Road Runners Club of America (RRCA)
1150 South Washington Street #250
Alexandria, VA 22314
Phone: (703) 836-0558
Fax: (703) 836-4430
e-mail: office@rrca.org
Web-Site: www.rrca.org

Senior Softball - USA Inc.
7052 Riverside Boulevard
Sacramento, CA 95831
Phone: (916) 393-8566
Fax: (916) 393-8350
Web-Site: www.seniorsoftball.com

Triathlon Federation/USA
3595 E. Fountain Boulevard, F-1
Colorado Springs, CO 80910
Phone: (719) 597-9090
Fax: (719) 597-2121
Web-Site: www.usatriathlon.org

USA Badminton
One Olympic Plaza
Colorado Springs, CO 80909
Phone: (719) 578-4808
Fax: (719) 578-4507
Web-Site: www.usabadminton.org

USA Karate Federation, Inc.
1300 Kenmore Boulevard
Akron, OH 44314
Phone: (330) 753-3114
Fax: (330) 753-6967
e-mail: usakf@raex.com
Web-Site: www.usakf.com

USA Table Tennis
One Olympic Plaza
Colorado Springs, CO 80909
Phone: (719) 578-4583
Fax: (719) 632-6071
Web-Site: www.usatt.org

USA Volleyball
3595 East Fountain Boulevard, Suite I-2
Colorado Springs, CO 80910
Phone: (719) 637-8300
Fax: (719) 597-6307
Web-Site: www.volleyball.org

United Square Dancers of America
8913 Seaton Drive
Huntsville, AL 35802
Phone: (205) 881-6044
Web-Site: cypress.idir.net/~usdanew

United States Aikido Federation
98 State Street
Northhampton, MA 01060
Phone and Fax: (413) 586-7122
Web-Site: www.usaikifed.org/usaf/home.html

United States Amateur Ballroom Dancers Association
P.O. Box 128
New Freedom, PA 17349
Phone: (800) 447-9047
Fax: (717) 235-4183
e-mail: usabdaccent@aol.com
Web-Site: www.world.std.com/~usabdant/

United States Amateur Confederation of Roller Skaters
4730 South
Lincoln, NE 68506
Phone: (402) 483-7551
Fax: (402) 483-1465
e-mail: usacrs@usacrs.com
Web-Site: www.usacrs.com

United States Cerebral Palsy Athletic Association
200 Harrison Avenue
Newport, RI 02840
Phone: (401) 848-2460
Fax: (401) 848-5280
e-mail: uscpaa@mail.bbsnet.com
Web-Site: www.uscpaa.org

United States Croquet Association
11585-B Polo Club Road
Wellington, FL 33414
Phone: (561) 753-9141
Fax: (561) 753-8801
e-mail: uscroquet@compuserve.com
Web-Site: www.ontheweb.com/usca

United States Field Hockey Association
One Olympic Plaza
Colorado Springs, CO 80909
Phone: (719) 578-4567
Fax: (719) 632-0979
Web-Site: www.usfieldhockey.com

United States Golf Association (USGA)
P.O. Box 708
Far Hills, NJ 07931
Phone: (908) 234-2300
Fax: (908) 234-9687
Web-Site: www.usga.org

United States Judo Association (USJA)
21 North Union Boulevard
Colorado Springs, CO 80919
Phone: (719) 633-7750
Fax: (719) 633-4041
Web-Site: www.csprings.com/usja

United States Masters Swimming
261 High Range Road
Londonderry, NH 03053-2616
Phone: (603) 537-0203
Fax: (603) 537-0204
e-mail: tracyswims@mindspring.com
Web-Site: www.usms.org

United States Professional Tennis Association
3535 Briarpark Drive
Houston, TX 77042
Phone: (713) 978-7782
Fax: (713) 978-7780
Web-Site: www.uspta.org

United States Rowing Association
201 South Capitol Avenue, Suite 400
Indianapolis, IN 46225
Phone: (317) 237-5656
Fax: (317) 237-5646
Web-Site: www.usrowing.org

United States Slo-Pitch Softball Association
3935 S. Crater Road
Petersburg, VA 23805
Phone: (804) 732-4099
Fax: (804) 732-1704
Web-Site: www.usssa.com

United States Squash Racquets Association (USSRA)
23 Cynwyd Road or P.O. Box 1216
Bala Cynwyd, PA 19004
Phone: (610) 667-4006
Fax: (610) 667-6539
Web-Site: www.us-squash.org/squash

United States Synchronized Swimming
201 South Capitol Avenue, Suite 901
Indianapolis, IN 46225
Phone: (317) 237-5700
Fax: (317) 237-5705
Web-Site: www.usasynchro.org

United States Tennis Association (USTA)
70 West Red Oak Lane
White Plains, NY 10604
Phone: (914) 696-7000
Fax: (914) 696-7167
e-mail: info@usta.com
Web-Site: www.usta.com

Wheelchair Sports, USA
3595 East Fountain Boulevard, Suite L-1
Colorado Springs, CO 80910
Phone: (719) 574-1150
Fax: (719) 574-9840
Web-Site: www.wsusa.org

World Masters Cross Country Ski Association
P.O. Box 5
Bend, OR 97709
Phone and Fax: (541) 382-3503
e-mail: dhuntwm@empnet.com

YMCA of the USA
101 North Wacker Drive
Chicago, IL 60606
Phone: (800) 872-9622
Fax: (312) 977-9063
Web-Site: www.ymca.net

YWCA of the USA
350 Fifth Avenue
New York City, NY 10118
Phone: (212) 273-7800
Fax: (212) 465-2281
Web-Site: www.ywca.org

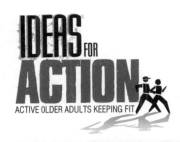

IDEAS FOR ACTION
ACTIVE OLDER ADULTS KEEPING FIT

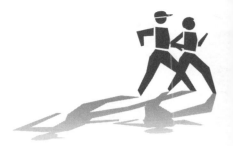

RESOURCE:

Associations & Organizations Offering Support Materials for Senior Fitness

American Association of Retired Persons (AARP)

Health & Long Term Care (HLTC)
601 E Street, NW
Washington, DC 20049
Phone: (202) 434-2230 or (202) 434-AARP
Fax: (202) 434-7683
Web-Site: www.aarp.org.

AARP is the nation's leading organization for people age 50 and over. It serves their needs and interests through legislative advocacy, research, informative programs and community services provided by a network of local chapters and experienced volunteers throughout the country. The organization also offers members a wide range of special membership benefits.

The AARP Health Advocacy Series offers a selection of resources concerning health and fitness. One such guide is *Activating Ideas: Promoting Physical Activity Among Older Adults*. This is a guide for Program Planners and Volunteer Leaders.

To obtain a catalog of available resources, call AARP Member Services at (800) 424-3410.

American College of Sports Medicine (ACSM)

401 W. Michigan Street
Indianapolis, IN 46202-3233
Phone: (317) 637-9200
Fax: (317) 634-7817
Web-Site: www.acsm.org/sportsmed

ACSM offers a variety of public education materials, including a "Fit Over 40" brochure outlining health and fitness considerations for those over 40 years of age.

They have been in existence since 1954 and have more than 16,000 members throughout the U.S. and around the world. There are 12 regional ACSM chapters in the U.S.

The American Parkinson Disease Association, Inc. (APDA)

1250 Hylan Boulevard, Suite 4B
Staten Island, NY 10305-1946
Phone: (718) 981-8001 or (800) 223-2732
Fax: (718) 981-4399
e-mail: APDA@ADMIN.CON2.COM
Web-Site: www.apdaparkinson.com

The American Parkinson Disease Association, Inc. was founded in 1961 to "Ease the Burden and Find the Cure" for Parkinson's disease and has been continuously growing ever since.

The APDA is the largest grass roots organization in the United States dedicated to fighting Parkinson's disease. The organization focuses its energies on research, patient service education, increased public awareness and patient advocacy.

The APDA offers a variety of educational booklets. *Be Active* is a 25-page booklet which details a suggested exercise program for people with Parkinson's disease. It is available in English, Italian and Japanese.

Center for the Study of Aging

706 Madison Avenue
Albany, NY 12208
Phone: (518) 465-6927
Fax: (518) 462-1339
Web-Site: members.aol.com/iapaas

The Center promotes education, research and training and provides leadership in the field of aging. In addition to ongoing consultant services in many fields, including mental and physical fitness, it conducts seminars and regional, national and international conferences, and maintains a 5,000-volume library.

Who? Me?! Exercise? – Safe Exercise for People Over 50 is a 40-page booklet with exercises and illustrations to help motivate and encourage all adults to exercise.

Cooper Institute for Aerobic Research
Cooper Fitness Center

12100 Preston Road
Dallas, TX 75230
Phone: (888) 964-8875 or (972) 233-4832
Fax: (972) 386-5760
Web-Site: www.cooperinst.org
Senior Fitness Consultant: Michel Kolling

The Cooper Institute for Aerobics Research, founded in 1970 by Dr. Ken Cooper, has become widely acclaimed as one of the leaders in preventive medicine *research* and *education*. As a non-profit research organization, The Cooper Institute is dedicated to advancing the understanding of the relationship between living habits and health and to providing leadership in implementing these concepts to enhance the *physical* and *emotional* well-being of individuals.

Training and certification programs for over 5,000 fitness leaders and health professionals are conducted annually. Programs are offered on our Dallas campus, at other sites throughout the U.S., and on a contract basis for organizations desiring specialized courses to meet unique needs.

A few of the senior-specific books available from the Cooper Institute include:

- *Fitness After 50* – A step by step guide for everyone over 50 who wants to be fit.

- *The Walking Handbook* – This handbook is ideal for walking clubs.

- *The Osteoporosis Handbook* – This book includes two illustrated exercise programs (for preventing and for treating).

- *Arthritis: Your Complete Exercise Guide*

- *Breathing Disorders: Your Complete Exercise Guide*

- *Diabetes: Your Complete Exercise Guide*

- *Stroke: Your Complete Exercise Guide*

Council on Aging and Adult Development (CAAD) - American Association for Active Lifestyles and Fitness (AAALF)

CAAD/AAALF
1900 Association Drive
Reston, VA 22091
Phone: (703) 476-3430
e-mail: aaalf@aahperd.org

The Council on Aging and Adult Development (CAAD) is a part of AAALF (American Association for Active Lifestyles and Fitness), one of six associations of the American Alliance for Health, Physical Education, Recreation and Dance (AAHPERD). It is one of the most active councils of AAALF, staying in the forefront of the information explosion related to physical activity programs for the older population. CAAD provides leadership in highly visible ways such as:

- Creation of a National Coalition of leading exercise associations to establish and publish a consensus of minimum competencies for senior exercise programs and instructors

- Publications promoting active lifestyles and fitness for older populations

- Training workshops for professionals and personnel working with older adults

- Latest information and research

Fifty-Plus Fitness Association

P.O. Box D
Stanford, CA 94309
Phone: (650) 323-6160
Fax: (650) 323-6119
e-mail: fitness@ix.netcom.com
Web-Site: www.50plus.org

The purpose of this association is to encourage fitness and a more active lifestyle for those who are fifty years or older, and to show that misuse and disuse of the body and mind are more the cause of disability than chronological age alone.

The mission of Fifty-Plus is to improve the physical fitness of older adults and to promote an active healthy lifestyle.

International Health, Racquet & Sportsclub Association (IHRSA)

263 Summer Street, Eighth Floor
Boston, MA 02210
Phone: (800) 228-4772
Fax: (617) 951-0056
e-mail: ihrsa@aol.com
Web-Site: www.ihrsa.org

Founded in 1981, IHRSA is a trade association for quality health clubs. Contact them for a list of health clubs in your area with programs for 50 and over.

NIA Alzheimer's Disease Education and Referral Center (ADEAR)

#NIAC, P.O. Box 8250
Silver Spring, MD 20907-8250
Phone: (800) 438-4380
Fax: (301) 495-3334
e-mail: adear@alzheimers.org
Web-Site: www.alzheimers.org/adear

National Association of Governor's Councils on Physical Fitness and Sports

201 S. Capitol Avenue, Suite 560
Indianapolis, IN 46255
Phone: (317) 237-5630
Fax: (317) 237-5632
e-mail: govcouncil@aol.com

The missions of the National Association of Governor's Council on Physical Fitness and Sports are to improve the quality of life for individuals in the United States through the promotion of physical fitness, sports involvement and healthy life styles and to foster and support Governor's Councils on Physical Fitness and Sports in every state and U.S. territory.

National Association of Senior Friends

P.O. Box 1300
Nashville, TN 37202-1300
Phone: (800) 348-4886
Fax: (615) 340-5757
Web-Site: www.columbia.net/senior/

Senior Friends is the largest healthcare based organization of adults 50 and over in the country. Started in 1986, Senior Friends has grown to over 222 chapters, all sponsored by Columbia hospitals, with more than 280,000 members.

Local chapters provide older adults with access to physical activity programs, workshops, instruction and classes.

National Institutes of Health National Institute on Aging

Building 31, Room 5C27
31 Center Drive MSC 2292
Bethesda, MD 20892-2292
Web-Site: www.nih.gov/nia

The National Institute on Aging (NIA) is one of the National Institutes of Health, the principal biomedical research agency of the United States government. The NIA promotes healthy aging by conducting and supporting biomedical, social, and behavioral research and public education.

The Public Information Office at the National Institute on Aging produces science-based educational materials on a wide range of topics related to health and aging including material on frailty and exercise and aging. Topics cover specific diseases and health conditions, treatments, and research. The materials are for use by the general public, patients and family members, health professionals, voluntary and community organizations, and the media. An on-line ordering form is available on the web-site.

For single copies, send the request by e-mail to: niainfo@access.digex.net or call toll-free (800) 222-2225 between 8:30 a.m and 5:00 p.m., EST.

Bulk orders can be filled upon request when inventory permits. Send written request by e-mail to: niainfo@access.digex.net, or write to the NIA Information Center at:

P.O. Box 8057
Gaithersburg, MD 20898-8057
Phone: (800) 222-2225
Fax: (301) 589-3014
e-mail: niainfo@access.digex.net

National Recreation and Parks Association (NRPA)

22377 Belmont Ridge Road
Ashburn, VA 20148
Phone: (703) 858-0784
Fax: (703) 858-0794
e-mail: info@nrpa.org
Web-Site: www.nrpa.org/

The National Recreation and Parks Association represents 4,500 parks and recreation facilities that offer programs in recreation and physical activity. The Leisure and Aging Section (LAS) of the NRPA unites professionals concerned about recreation and leisure services for older adults who are employed by municipal park and recreation agencies and retirement communities.

Publications from the NRPA include:

- *Best Practice Programs in Leisure and Aging* – this manual describes eight unique and excellent programs offered from across the nation and includes detailed information about each program in an easy to replicate format

- *Dynamic Leisure Programming with Older Adults* – this collection of articles includes information on leisure participation in retirement communities, wellness programs, recreation for frail older adults, programming in long term care facilities, and management of senior centers.

For more information and to get a list of other available publications, contact the Leisure and Aging Section staff liaison at (703) 858-0784.

National Wellness Institute, Inc.

1300 College Court
P.O. Box 827
Stevens Point, WI 54481-0827
Phone: (715) 342-2969
Fax: (715) 342-2979
e-mail: nwi@wellnessnwi.org
Web-Site: www.wellnessnwi.org/

A non-profit corporation committed to the promotion of optimal well-being. National Wellness Institute's (NWI) mission is accomplished through national and international leadership via professional education conferences, a membership division, and the development and distribution of wellness-related products and services.

President's Council on Physical Fitness and Sports (PCPFS)

200 Independence Avenue SW
HHH Building, Room 738H
Washington, DC 20201
Phone: (202) 690-9000
Fax: (202) 690-5211
Web-Site:
    www.os.dhhs.gov/progorg/ophs/pcpfs.htm

Founded in 1956, the President's Council on Physical Fitness and Sports promotes participation in physical fitness and sports for all Americans. One of their major functions is information dissemination and public awareness about the importance of physical activity and fitness.

Two areas in which the PCPFS promotes fitness in the senior population are:

• Silver Eagle Corp

• President's Sports Award Program.

Sporting Goods Manufacturers Association (SGMA) Sports Apparel Products Council

200 Castlewood Drive
North Palm Beach, FL 33408
Phone: (561) 840-1151
Fax: (561) 863-8984
Web-Site: www.sportlink.com/sport

• The SGMA developed the *Active & Ageless Resource Guide* to help people easily locate physical fitness activities where they live, work and travel. The comprehensive 200-page soft-covered directory includes more than 1,000 listings of local groups and national organizations with fitness programs for persons over age 50.

• *Let's Get Moving* contains information about physical activity for women over age 50.

Both of these resources can be purchased from the SGMA while supplies last.

Surgeon General's Report on Physical Activity and Health

Information on the Surgeon General's Report on Physical Activity and Health is available on the Centers for Disease Control and Prevention's web page at: www.cdc.gov/whatsnew.htm

Additional information on the SGR can be found on the Sporting Goods Manufacturer's Association (SGMA) web-site at: www.sportlink.com/fitness

Other Support Organizations:

American Cancer Society
1599 Clifton Road, N.E.
Atlanta, GA 30329-4251
Phone: (800) 227-2345
Web-Site: www.cancer.org

American Diabetes Association
1660 Duke Street
Alexandria, VA 22314
Phone: (800) 232-3472
Fax: (703) 549-6995
Web-Site: www.diabetes.org

American Dietetic Association
216 W. Jackson Boulevard
Chicago, IL 60606-6995
Phone: (312) 899-0040
Fax: (312) 899-1979
Web-Site: www.eatright.org

The American Geriatrics Society
770 Lexington Avenue, Suite 300
New York City, NY 10021
Phone: (212) 308-1414
Fax: (212) 832-8646
Web-Site: www.americangeriatrics.org

American Heart Association (AHA)
7272 Greenville Avenue
Dallas, TX 75231
Phone: (800) 242-1793
Web-Site: www.amhrt.org/

American Lung Association (ALA)
1740 Broadway
New York City, NY 10019
Phone: (212) 315-8700
Fax: (212) 315-8872
Web-Site: www.lungusa.org

Arthritis Foundation
1330 W. Peachtree Street
Atlanta, GA 30309
Phone: (800) 283-7800
Fax: (404) 872-0457
Web-Site: www.arthritis.org

Foundation for Glaucoma Research
490 Post Street, Suite 830
San Francisco, CA 94102-9950
Phone: (415) 986-3162
Fax: (415) 986-3763
Web-Site: www.glaucoma.org

Healthwise
2601 N. Bogus Basin Road
Boise, ID 83702
Phone: (208) 345-1161
Fax: (208) 345-1897
Web-Site: www.healthwise.org

National Arthritis, Musculoskeletal, and
  Skin Disease Information Clearinghouse
9000 Rockville Pike, Box AMS
Bethesda, MD 20892
Phone: (301) 495-4484
Fax: (301) 587-4352
Web-Site: www.nih.gov/niams

National Center for Health Statistics
  Statistical Resources Branch
  Division of Vital Statistics
6525 Belcrest Road, Room 820
Hyattsville, MD 20782
Phone: (301) 436-8979
Fax: (301) 436-7066
Web-Site:
  www.cdc.gov/nchswww/about/major/dvs/
  mordata.htm

National Council on the Aging, Inc. (NCOA)
409 Third Street, SW, Second Floor
Washington, DC 20024
Phone: (202) 479-1200
Fax: (202) 479-0735
Web-Site: www.ncoa.org

National Health Information Center
P.O. Box 1133
Washington, DC 20013-1133
Phone: (800) 336-4797
Fax: (301) 468-3028
e-mail: nhicinfo@health.org
Web-Site: nhic-nt.health.org

National Heart, Lung, and Blood Institute
P.O. Box 30105
Bethesda, MD 20824-0105
Phone: (301) 251-1222
Fax: (301) 251-1223
Web-Site: www.nih.gov

National Mental Health Association (NMHA)
1021 Prince Street
Alexandria, VA 22314-2971
Phone: (703) 684-7722
Fax: (703) 684-5968
Web-Site: www.nmha.org

National Osteoporosis Foundation
1150 17th Street, NW, Suite 500
Washington, DC 20036
Phone: (202) 223-2226
Fax: (202) 223-2237
Web-Site: www.nof.org

National Safety Council
1121 Spring Lake Drive
Itasca, IL 60143-3201
Phone (800) 621-7619
Fax: (630) 285-0797
Web-Site: www.nsc.org

National Stroke Association
96 Inverness Drive East, Suite I
Englewood, CO 80112
Phone: (303) 649-9299
Fax: (303) 649-1328
Web-Site: www.stroke.org

Prostate Health Council
c/o American Foundation for Urologic
Disease, Inc.
1128 North Charles Street
Baltimore, MD 21201
Phone: (800) 242-2383
Fax: (410) 468-1808
Web-Site: www.afud.org

Self-Help for Hard of Hearing People, Inc.
7910 Woodmont Avenue, Suite 1200
Bethesda, MD 20814
Phone: (301) 657-2248
Fax: (301) 913-9413
e-mail: national@shhh.org
Web-Site: www.shhh.org

U.S. Department of Agriculture, Food
and Nutrition Information Center
National Agricultural Library
10301 Baltimore Avenue, Room 304
Beltsville, MD 20705
Phone: (301) 504-5719
Web-Site: www.nal.usda.gov/fnic

Wellness Councils of America
7101 Newport Avenue, Suite 311
Omaha, NE 68152
Phone: (402) 572-3590
Fax: (402) 572-3594
e-mail: welcoa@neonramp.com
Web-Site: www.welcoa.org

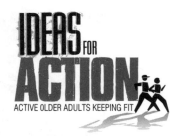

IDEAS FOR
ACTION
ACTIVE OLDER ADULTS KEEPING FIT

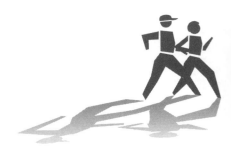

Body Recall, Inc.

Body Recall, Inc.
P.O. Box 412
Berea, KY 40403
Phone: (606) 986-2181
Fax: (606) 986-7580

Program Description

Body Recall is a nonprofit, non-franchised, nationwide exercise program. The program is conducted by certified teachers in hospitals, retirement homes, YMCA's, parks and recreation centers, senior citizen centers, community colleges, churches, health clubs and on college campuses. Contact Body Recall for information on training and workshops.

Publications and programs for seniors:

Body Recall, A Program of Physical Fitness for the Adult is a 208-page large-print book which includes exercises on range of motion and strength that can be done sitting, standing or lying down. It also contains information on body mechanics, foot care, falls and recovery techniques.

Week-long teacher training in Body Recall is available throughout the year in Berea, Kentucky. Special populations training and certification are available.

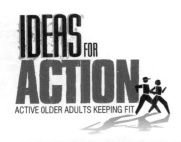

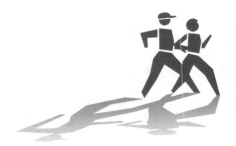

IDEAS FOR ACTION
ACTIVE OLDER ADULTS KEEPING FIT

Collage Video Guide

Collage Video
5390 Main Street NE
Minneapolis, MN 55421-1128

Phone: (612) 571-5840 or (800) 433-6769
Fax: (612) 571-5906
Web-Site: www.collagevideo.com

Guide Objective

To provide accurate information on a wide variety of exercise videos

Program Description

Before any video can be considered for this catalog, it's done by two people (a certified staff instructor who looks for technique and a "regular" person who rates it for motivation/interest).

Videos are then listed in the guide using a consistent format which provides information concerning exercise level, color-coded exercise breakdown and style of video.

Table of Contents:
- Aerobics
- Muscle Toning
- Aerobics & Toning
- Stretch & Mind/Body

Additional Specialty Workouts include:
- Seniors
- Back Pain
- Special Situations
- Kids
- Pregnancy

The "Sit and Be Fit" series is just one of the listings found in the Senior Workout section. It features six separate videos for six distinct physical conditions which include:

- Stroke
- Chronic Obstructive Pulmonary Disease
- Multiple Sclerosis
- Parkinson's
- Osteoporosis
- Arthritis

Procedure

Many of the videos listed in this guide are not available in stores.

To obtain an issue of *The Complete Guide to Exercise Videos* call 1 (800) 433-6769.

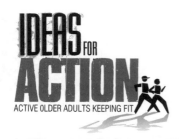

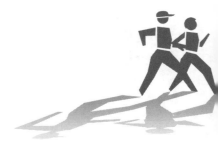

Companies Offering Products or Resources for Senior Fitness

Aquatic Trends, Inc.

649 U.S. Hwy. One, Suite 14
North Palm Beach, FL 33408
Phone: (800) 296-5496 or (561) 844-3003
Fax: (561) 844-0302
e-mail: aquatictrends@flinet.com
Web-Site: www.aquatictrends.com

The AQUATREND "Water Workout Station" uses water to provide a health maintenance and rehabilitation program. The "Water Workout Station" offers a total body workout regardless of age or physical condition. It is easy to install and can be removed and stored. It is recommended by doctors, physical therapists and aquatic experts. The AQUATREND approach offers a variety of exercise options such as toning, strengthening, rehabilitative care, cardiovascular conditioning, weight loss and relief for people suffering from arthritis.

A newsletter entitled "AQUA-TREND ADVISOR" is provided to share information concerning the "station" and provide protocol for various users.

For more information on the "Water Workout Station" and to order a free video, call (800) 296-5496.

Keiser Sports Health Equipment

411 S. West Avenue
Fresno, CA 93706-1320
Phone: (800) 888-7009 or (209) 265-4700
Fax: (209) 265-4760
Web-Site: www.keiser.com
Contact: Dennis Keiser

Since 1990, Keiser has been considered the leading manufacturer in research on aging. The Keiser air-power design allows the user to increase resistance in single-pound increments.

Keiser continues to support both education and programming in the area of mature-adult fitness. Keiser is a sponsor of the International Conference on Aging and Physical Activity and is also the sponsor of the International Health Racquet and Sportsclub Association (IHRSA)/Keiser 50 Plus award for best mature-adult fitness programs.

The future sees Keiser continuing to be heavily involved in research on reversing the effects of aging.

Contact them for more information about research and program design.

LifePlus, Inc.

3770 Plaza Drive, Suite 1
Ann Arbor, MI 48108
Phone: (800) 322-2209
Fax: (313) 769-8180

The NuStep Total Body Recumbent Steppers have proven to be an important component to many senior fitness programs. Their unique design allows for a variety of users with a multitude of health concerns.

The LIFE*Plus* Newsletter is a wealth of information about exercise and aging.

Contact them for more information.

Star Trac

14352 Chambers Road
Tustin, CA 92780
Phone: (800) 228-6635 or (714) 669-1660
Fax: (714) 838-6286
Web-Site: www.startrac.com

Star Trac, a manufacturer of aerobic products, has introduced support materials which can be used with a mature adult population. These materials are designed to be used as an educational tool to support programming efforts.

Materials include:

- *Delay the Onset of Aging* – a look at how America's population is aging and the challenges it brings to all fitness professionals; solutions to these challenges are included

- *Walk it Off!* – a 12-week program designed to attract participants who would not typically join a fitness facility

- *Weight Management* – lifelong weight management can be achieved only through lifestyle change – healthy lifestyle solutions are offered

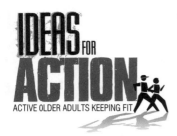

IDEAS FOR ACTION

ACTIVE OLDER ADULTS KEEPING FIT

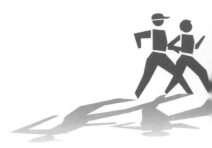

RESOURCE:

Creative Walking, Inc.

Creative Walking, Inc.
P.O. Box 50296
Clayton, MO 63105

Phone: (800) 762-9255
Fax: (314) 721-0303

Program Description

Author and Creative Walking, Inc. developer Rob Sweetgall has walked across America seven times since 1982, including a 50-state walk of 11,208 miles in one year. Author of numerous books on walking and wellness, Rob has presented motivational workshops and seminars to over 500,000 people worldwide. The Walking Wellness curriculum he developed is now used by thousands of individuals in all 50 states.

Books available from Creative Walking, Inc. include:

- *Fitness Walking*
- *The Walker's Journal*
- *Treadmill Walking*
- *Road Scholars*
- *Walking Off Weight*

For more information, contact Creative Walking, Inc. at the address above.

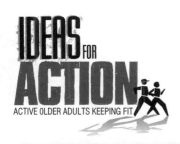

IDEAS FOR ACTION
ACTIVE OLDER ADULTS KEEPING FIT

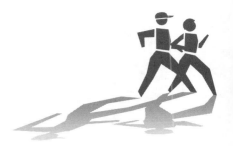

Fitness Educators of Older Adults Association (FEOAA)

Fitness Educators of Older Adults Association (FEOAA)
759 Chopin Drive, Suite 1
Sunnyvale, CA 94087
Phone: (408) 450-1224
Contact: Dr. Karl G. Knopf, Executive Director

Organization Description

FEOAA is a nonprofit organization which addresses the health and wellness concerns of the older adult population. FEOAA holds healthy aging workshops throughout the country and publishes quarterly newsletters addressing various health issues relative to the adult population. FEOAA also trains professionals such as fitness trainers, nursing home staff and medical personnel who work with the adult community.

Workshops offered include:

- **Healthy Aging Workshop** – this workshop is designed to provide the instructor of Older Adult Exercise Classes the most up-to-date knowledge and techniques available to be the best teacher possible. Topics include "What's Age Got To Do With It?," "Special Populations," "Gero-Kinesiology" and "Putting It All Together."

- **The Adaptive Fitness Instructor/Special Population Workshop** – topics include "Care and Prevention of Back Disorders," "Exercise Prescription and Chronic Conditions," "Water Exercise and the Disabled" and "How to Design an Exercise Program for the Disabled."

- **Fit For Life Wellness Weekend** is a workshop designed for mature adults and provides educational fitness/wellness information. Participants receive quarterly newsletters containing useful and accurate information written expressly for mature adults. Topics include "Exercise Do's and Don'ts," "How to Get and Stay Fit Tips," and reviews of books, videos and products designed for older adults.

FEOAA Bookstore

Videos:
- *Over Sixty and Feeling Fit*
- *How to Teach the Older Adult*

Books:
- *Fitness Over Fifty*
- *Water Workouts*
- *Adaptive Physical Education for the Adult with Disabilities*

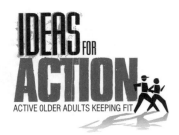

ACTIVE OLDER ADULTS KEEPING FIT

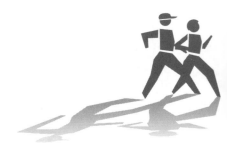

IDEA Educational Products Catalog

International Association of Fitness Professionals (IDEA)
6190 Cornerstone Court E., Suite 204
San Diego, CA 92121-4701
Phone: (800) 999-4332 ext. 7 or (619) 535-8979 ext. 7
Fax: (619) 535-8234
Web-Site: www.ideafit.com

Organization Description

IDEA was founded in 1982 and is dedicated solely to meeting the specific needs of fitness professionals, aerobics instructors, personal trainers, club owners, managers and program directors.

Catalog Description

The IDEA Educational Products Catalog contains information on:

- Independent Study Courses
- Audiotapes
- Videotapes
- Booklets

Categories in this catalog include:
- Choreography
- Strength/Resistance Training
- Personal Training
- Weight Management
- Exercise Science
- Special Populations
- Water Fitness
- Attracting and Motivating Clients
- Consumer Pamphlets

The **Special Population - Aging** Category includes the following selections:

- *Exercise Testing, Exercise Prescription and Safety Concerns for Working with Older Clients* – This course shows you how to modify a fitness program for frail adults.

- *Program Design for Special Populations* – This course presents the medical concerns of special populations and their implications for your exercise programming.

- *Exercise for the 50+ Adult* – Offers proven strategies for marketing to and programming for "Baby Boomers." Explains the physiology of older adults and provides recommendations on music that will add fun to your senior workouts.

- *Exercise and Aging* – This audio tape explains the special health, mobility and programming issues to consider when designing exercise programs for older adults.

- *Exercise, Aging and Menopause* – Explores the effects of aging on aerobic capacity, muscular strength, bone density, lean body mass and other factors. This tape outlines the major problems women face with menopause.

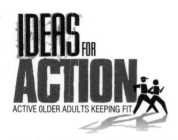

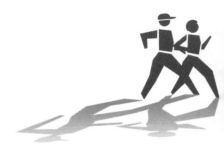

RESOURCE:

Jazzercise, Inc.

Jazzercise, Inc.
2808 Roosevelt Street
Carlsbad, CA 92008
Phone: (760) 434-2101 or (800) FIT-IS-IT
Fax: (760) 434-8958
Web-Site: www.jazzercise.com

Organization Objective

To offer exercise classes for individuals with a wide range of abilities and fitness levels

Program Description

Jazzercise LITE

This low intensity format, for a low to moderate level of workout, is designed for individuals with health considerations, such as beginning exercisers, senior citizens or those who simply want to enjoy a moderate workout. Movements can be done at a more intense level if desired by the individual exerciser.

Musical Chairs

This musically active class incorporates simple resistance exercises using rubber tubing and light free weights (for strength) with stylized walking patterns (for cardiovascular conditioning.) The choreography is simple and the muscle work can be done seated, which decreases balance difficulties. This class is FUN and EASY to do for all ages and is especially popular with those who are new to exercise or wishing to maintain workouts during a time when lighter workouts are needed.

Other Jazzercise class formats include:

- jazzercise
- jazzercise plus
- simply jazzercise
- body sculpting jazzercise
- cardio quick jazzercise
- circuit training jazzercise
- step by jazzercise
- personal touch jazzercise

Procedure

For more information on class locations, instructors or certification call (800) FIT-IS-IT or (760) 434-2101. Visit the Jazzercise web-site at www.jazzercise.com and click on "Corporate Information" or "Class Information" and then "Become an Instructor."

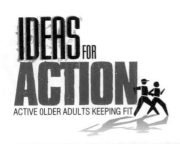

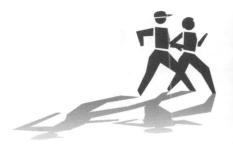

RESOURCE:

National Senior Health & Fitness Day (NSHFD)

National Senior Health & Fitness Day
Mature Market Resource Center
621 East Park Avenue
Libertyville, IL 60048

Phone: (800) 828-8225
Fax: (847) 816-8662
e-mail: maturemkt@aol.com

Program Description

Organized as a public/private partnership by the Mature Market Resource Center (MMRC), National Senior Health & Fitness Day (NSHFD) will offer fitness activities for adults in senior centers, park and recreation departments, hospitals, retirement communities, houses of worship, banks and other community locations. The event is always held on the last Wednesday in May as part of Older Americans Month celebrations.

Last year, programs ranged from small group exercise sessions in community senior centers to walking tours and outdoor health fairs. Most programs include an exercise or physical activity component, as well as educational information about senior health and fitness.

To help older adults stay motivated after National Senior Health & Fitness Day, the MMRC created the Mature Fitness Awards USA, the nation's first fitness recognition program solely for older adults. This unique awards program is open to adults age 50 and over, and recognizes older adult fitness achievements in a wide variety of physical activities such as aerobics, bicycling, group exercise, swimming and walking. Individuals can earn the award annually.

Contact the Mature Market Resource Center for more information on the upcoming National Senior Health & Fitness Day and the Mature Fitness Awards USA.

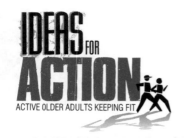

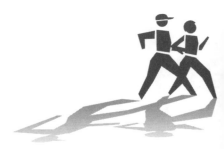

RESOURCE:

Senior Fitness Consultants

Don Callahan
Keiser Sports Health Equipment
31 Millbrook Road
Wayland, MA 01778
Phone: (888) 544-9844 or (508) 358-5993
Fax: (508) 358-5282

Janie T. Clark, M.S., President
American Senior Fitness Association
P.O. Box 2575
New Smyrna Beach, FL 32170
Phone: (904) 423-6634
Fax: (904) 427-0613

Gary Eippert, Ph.D, President
The Wellness Advisor, Inc.
9 McCormick Trail
Milford, OH 45150
Phone & Fax: (513) 576-1409

Dennis Keiser
Keiser Sports Health Equipment
411 S. West Avenue
Fresno, CA 93706-1320
Phone: (800) 683-1236
Fax: (209) 265-4760
Web-Site: www.keiser.com

Karl Knopf, Ed.D
Fitness Educators of Older Adults
   Association
759 Chopin Drive, Suite 1
Sunnyvale, CA 94087
Phone: (408) 735-9398

Linda Mazie, M.Ed., President
Partners in Fitness, Inc.
7 Gibson Avenue
Dedham, MA 02026
Phone: (781) 326-6917
Fax: (781) 326-3107
e-mail: pifinc@aol.com

Jan Montague, MGS, Director
Wellness Center
Maple Knoll Village
11100 Springfield Pike
Cincinnati, OH 45246
Phone: (513) 782-4340

Wayne H. Osness, Ph.D.
Department of Health, Sports, and
   Exercise Sciences
161 Robinson Center
Lawrence, KS 66045-2348
Phone: (785) 864-5482
Fax: (785) 864-3343
e-mail: waosn@falcon.cc.ukans.edu

John Rude, President
John Rude & Associates
2749 Friendly Street, Suite D
Eugene, OR 97405
Phone: (800) 929-2719
Fax: (541) 343-3697
e-mail: info@agedynamics.com
Web-Site: agedynamics.com

Kay Van Norman
SenioRS Unlimited
7880 Fowler Lane
Bozeman, MT 59717
Phone: (406) 587-0786
e-mail: Kayvn@montana.campus.mci.net

Jerry & Donna Yost
MaxLife Fitness Center Directors
Robson Communities
9532 East Riggs Road
Sun Lakes, AZ 85248
Phone: (800) 223-7317 or (602) 802-6853
Fax: (602) 802-2622

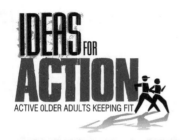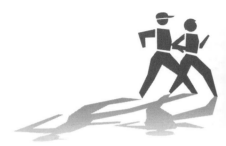

IDEAS FOR ACTION
ACTIVE OLDER ADULTS KEEPING FIT

Senior Fitness Videos & Books

Video, Music and Audio Tapes

Aerobic Beat Music Co. (Ken Alan Associates)
7985 Santa Monica Boulevard, Suite 109
Los Angeles, CA 90046-5186
Phone: (213) 653-5040
Fax: (213) 655-5223

- *Age is the Rage: Part 1* video includes an educational discussion on significant social and physiological issues associated with aging, and offers recommendations for meeting the exercise and activity needs of older adults.

- *Age is the Rage: Part 2* video includes creative model workouts and offers helpful tips for instructors.

- *Senior Workout 4* is a music tape especially designed for use with older adult groups, but it is not old-fashioned.

Aviano USA
1199 Avenida Acaso, Suite K
Camarillo, CA 93012
Phone: (805) 484-8138

- *Rise Up With Rosie* is a 55-minute video of exercise and dance rhythms for older adults, featuring motivational senior specialist Rose P. Metter. Part one is "Chair Exercises" and part two is "Rhythm Time."

- *Keep Fit While You Sit* is a video catering to people who wish to exercise while seated.

CC-M Productions
8510 Cedar Street
Silver Springs, MD 20910
Phone: (800) 453-6280
Fax: (301) 585-2321
e-mail: cc-m@cc-m.com

- *Armchair Fitness Aerobics* is an aerobic workout in a chair for those who, because of preference, lifestyle, age or disability, need or want to avoid vigorous activity.

- *Armchair Fitness Gentle Exercise* is a program for persons with limited strength and range of motion.

- *Armchair Fitness Strength Improvement* is a two-session program which includes aerobic, strength building with neckties, and upper body strengthening using soup cans as weights.

- *Armchair Fitness Yoga* includes three sessions: breathing for relaxation, coordinated stretching and yoga movements in a chair.

Cottonwood Press
305 West Magnolia, Suite 398
Ft. Collins, CO 80521
Phone: (800) 864-4297
Web Site: www.verinet.com/cottonwood

- *Exercise SeniorStyle* video features two exercise sessions. Session One features primarily seated exercises and Session Two has more standing exercises. Workouts are designed to improve flexibility, strength and overall fitness.

Downtown Atlanta Senior Services
607 Peachtree Street
Atlanta, GA 30365
Phone: (404) 872-9191

- *Stay Fit for Life* shows an exercise program for adults over age 50. The program was developed by gerontological health and fitness professionals.

- *Active for Life* is a special training program for those working with long-term care patients and the frail elderly.

Dynamix Music Service
733 W. 40th, Suite 10
Baltimore, MD 21211
Phone: (410) 243-9755 or (800) 843-6499

Elder Books
P.O. Box 490
Forest Knolls, CA 94933
Phone: (415) 488-9002
Fax: (415) 488-4720

- *Music, Movement, Mind, Body* is a dementia-specific physical activity program. This new music and exercise program was developed specifically for persons with Alzheimer's disease and related disorders. The kit, which includes an audio music tape and accompanying booklet, is a great resource for activity personnel working in long term care

settings. Although the program was initially designed for persons with dementia, it has also been used successfully with persons affected by other conditions, such as stroke.

Fitwise Productions, Inc.
P.O. Box 759
Jericho, NY 11753

- *Seniorobics*
  This is actually a book, but it comes with a workout music tape. Readers can do the workout given in the book along with the music provided. Write for a brochure.

Gunderson Lutheran Medical Center
1919 South Avenue
La Crosse, WI 54601-9980
Phone: (800) 362-9567, ext. 4787

- *Swing into Shape* is a low-intensity, nonaerobic exercise video program that includes three exercise routines which progress in intensity. The program is designed especially for use by older adults and those with physical limitations.

Kimbo Educational
P.O. Box 477
Long Branch, NJ 07740
Phone: (732) 229-4949
Fax: (732) 870-3340

- *Fitness for Seniors*, an audio cassette, offers several routines for the older adult. Each musical routine moves through a sequence of movements from warm-up to recharge.

- *Seatworks* and *Sittercise* are both available as an audio cassette and provide a musical seated workout for a wide range of ages and capabilities. Each cassette is accompanied by a manual giving specific suggestions for use with older adults, as well as written instructions and illustrations of the exercises.

Power Music

1303 S. Swaner Road
Salt Lake City, UT 84104-4115
Phone: (800) 777-2328

ProMotion Music

1611 North Stemmons, Suite 416
Carrollton, TX 75006
Phone: (800) 380-4776 or (972) 446-0388

Sit and Be Fit, Inc.

P.O. Box 8033
Spokane, WA 99203-0033
Phone: (509) 448-9438

Chair exercise programs for adults 50 years and older, as well as individuals with physical limitations. Professionally designed by Mary Ann Wilson, RN, this program truly helps people become functionally fit again and improve their quality of life.

Video and audio tapes focus on balancing the body – stretching tight muscles and strengthening weak ones. A list of applicable participants includes people recovering from strokes and heart attacks, those with chronic conditions such as arthritis, multiple sclerosis, respiratory ailments and injured individuals experiencing the slow process of rehabilitation.

Sports Music

Box 769689
Roswell, GA 30076
Phone: (800) 878-4764
Fax: (770) 664-4557

V.I.E.W. Video, Inc.

34 East 23rd Street
New York City, NY 10010
Phone: (212) 674-5550
Fax: (212) 979-0266

- *Exercise Can Beat Arthritis* was developed by a physical therapist who works with the Arthritis Foundation. The video's exercise participants include a variety of people who actually have arthritis. No resistance exercise is included, and the cardiovascular segment is short, consisting of low-intensity, mainly chair-supported activities.

Wheelchair Workout

12275 Greenleaf Avenue
Potomac, MD 20854
Phone: (301) 279-2994

- *Wheelchair Workout with Janet Reed* includes an audio cassette tape and a 43-page manual providing a program of upper body exercises which can be done from a wheelchair, a sturdy chair or while standing. The manual includes illustrations and instructions for each exercise.

- *Fitness and Independence with Janet Reed,* a 14-minute motivational video which illustrates upper body exercises and encourages fitness for people in wheelchairs.

Books

Aging, Physical Activity, and Health

By Roy J. Shepherd
Published by Human Kinetics

The Arthritis Exercise Book

By Gwen Ellert
Published by Contemporary Books

Good exercise advice for those with arthritis. Easy to understand. Large print. Can be ordered through bookstores.

Be Alive as Long as You Live

By Lawrence J. Frankel and
  Betty Byrd Richard
Published by Lippincott & Crowell, NY

Includes simple, easy-to-learn exercises to help strengthen heart and lungs, tone muscles, and increase flexibility. A helpful guide for use at home by older persons or for conducting simple exercise programs for those who are physically more limited.

Biomarkers: The 10 Keys to Prolonging Vitality

By William J. Evans, Ph.D. and
  Irwin H. Rosenberg, M.D.

This book looks into research from the USDA Human Nutrition Research Center on Aging at Tufts University, which demonstrates the body's decline is due *not* to the passing of years but to the combined effects of inactivity, poor nutrition and illness. The authors have identified ten "biomarkers," the key physiological factors associated with prolonged youth and vitality.

Body Recall
By Dorothy Chrisman
Published by Human Kinetics

Chair Exercise Manual

By Eva Desca Garnet
Published by Princeton Book Company,
   Princeton, NJ

Offers techniques, and chair exercises emerging from them, which have been tested by Ms. Garnet in classroom and hospital situations. For those with more limited physical ability. Available with audio-cassette.

Complete Guide to Aging & Health

By Mark E. Williams, M.D.
Published by the American Geriatrics
   Society (212) 308-1414

The book contains expert advice for those who wish to prepare for a healthy old age, as well as for those who are involved in the care of older individuals. Topics covered in this book include changes that occur as our bodies and minds age and prevention strategies.

The Cooper Clinic and Research Institute Fitness Series

By Neil Gordon
Published by Human Kinetics

This is a series of five exercise guidebooks for persons with diabetes, chronic fatigue, breathing disorders, arthritis, and history of stroke. Can be ordered through bookstores.

Elder Fit: A Health and Fitness Program for Older Adults

By Diane Penner
Published by AAPHERD Publications
   (800) 321-0789

A comprehensive exercise and fitness program for frail elderly with eight pre-planned exercise sessions.

Exercise and the Older Adult

By Wayne Osness
Published by AAPHERD Publications
   (800) 321-0789

This is the prime textbook in the field including biomechanics, exercise physiology and motor learning of aging. Activity planning includes sitting, as well as aquatic exercise and dance.

Exercise for Older Adults

By American Council on Exercise
Published by Human Kinetics

Exercise Programming for Older Adults

Edited by Janie Clark, M.S.
Published by the Haworth Press

Published in April of 1996, this excellent resource includes chapters written by highly respected experts on aerobics, strength training, stretching, posture and breathing exercises, stroke management and hot water exercise therapy. It is particularly recommended for activity directors in long term care settings such as nursing homes and adult day care centers.

Exercise Programming for Older Adults

By Kay A. Van Norman
Published by Human Kinetics

This book provides everything you need in order to develop, market and manage a fitness program for older adults. It's a valuable resource for health/fitness instructors, recreation specialists and facility directors who want to learn how to meet the needs of the growing seniors market. Can be ordered through bookstores.

Fitness for Life

By Charels B. Corbin and Ruth Lindsey
Published by Human Kinetics

Forever Fit – The Exercise Program for Staying Young

By Morton D. Bogdonoff, M.D.
Published by Little, Brown and Co., Boston

Includes suggestions for those who have heart ailments, back problems and respiratory diseases. Directed at a general older readership.

Full Life Fitness
By Janie Clark, M.S.
Published by Human Kinetics

An excellent, complete fitness program for mature adults. Includes many illustrations and helpful exercise tips. Covers low impact aerobic dance, muscle conditioning exercises, stretching, swimming pool exercise and active leisure pastimes. Can be ordered through bookstores.

Functional Fitness Assessment For Adults Over 60 Years (A Field Based Assessment) Second Edition
By Wayne H. Osness, Marlene Adrian, Bruce Clark, Werner Hoeger, Diane Raab and Robert Wiswell
Published by Kendall/Hunt, Dubuque, Iowa

The functional fitness assessment of adults over 60 years of age is important in evaluating the ability of the individual to carry on certain daily living activities and, even more important, as one contemplates a physical training or rehabilitation program intended to help the individual improve their functional capacity over time. This manual explains the assessment procedures that have been designed to serve the larger population through field based measurement techniques that can be used in a facility where older persons live, and can be conducted by personnel not necessarily trained for clinical responsibilities. (Companion video to this manual which demonstrates each item and gives tips on what to look for with various conditions is available from AAHPERD Publications at (800) 321-0789.)

Guide to Fitness After 50
By Raymond Harris, M.D. and Lawrence Frankel, Eds.
Published by Plenum Press, NY

Presents basic and applied research data, authoritative advice, and tested techniques for professional workers and other individuals who want to learn more about physical exercise, fitness and relaxation for older people.

Maximizing Options for a Quality Life
Published by AAPHERD Publications (800) 321-0789

This informative pamphlet represents CAAD's position on the professional standards that should be met by facilities offering programs for seniors.

Physical Dimensions of Aging
By Waneen W. Spirduso, Ed.D.
Published by Human Kinetics

While the field of aging is notable for its rich collections of data, it has also suffered from a general lack of integration. But with the publication of *Physical Dimensions of Aging*, that is no longer the case. Not only does Dr. Spirduso thoroughly review the facts about physical aging, but more important, she synthesizes those facts in a coherent story that reveals how our bodies age.

Research Sourcebook and Bibliography in Aging and Health, Exercise, Recreation and Dance
By Charlie Daniel, Veronica Eskridge, Linda D. Frizzll, and Dean Gorman
Published by AAPHERD Publications (800) 321-0789

A ready-made bibliography of current publications in exercise and aging. It also includes listing of private foundations and other funding sources.

Seniors on the Move
By Renate Rikkers
Published by Human Kinetics

A sensitively written guide for fitness instructors in search of practical ideas and current information on designing programs for seniors. Can be ordered through bookstores.

Seniorcise: A Simple Guide to Fitness for the Elderly and Disabled

By Janie Clark, M.S.
Published by Pineapple Press, Inc.

Strength Training Past 50

By Wayne Westcott and Thomas R. Baechle
Published by Human Kinetics

Therapeutic Dance/Movement Expressive Activities for Older Adults

By Erna Caplow-Lindner, Leah Harpaz
and Sonya Samberg
Published by Human Sciences Press, NY

Provides professionals with guidelines and specific material to conduct therapeutic movement sessions. Integrates creative and folk dance movements, yoga, and standard exercises especially adapted to the limited coordination and strength of the elderly.

We Live Too Short and Die Too Long

By Walter M. Bortz II, M.D.
Published by Bantam Books

In this ground-breaking work, Dr. Bortz sets out the essential, controllable elements of longevity and spells out effective, dynamic strategies to help you prevent premature death and add decades of active, satisfying life. He outlines the basic practices *you can start today* – no matter what your age. Available in bookstores.

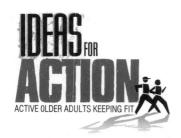

ACTIVE OLDER ADULTS KEEPING FIT

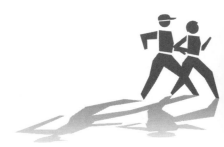

RESOURCE:

U.S. Water Fitness Association

U.S. Water Fitness Association (USWFA)
P.O. Box 3279
Boynton Beach, FL 33424-3279

Phone: (561) 732-9908
Fax: (561) 732-0950
e-mail: uswfa@emi.net
Web-Site: www.emi.net/~uswfa/

Program Description

The U.S. Water Fitness Association believes that "water exercise is for everyone!"

Reasons why exercising *in* the water is better than exercising *out* of the water:

1. **Buoyancy:** The water property allows people to do exercises that are difficult to do on land. 90% of your body is buoyant when in the water up to your neck, so you are not hitting the floor as hard as you would on land, therefore no pounding or jarring is felt.

2. **Resistance:** There is continual resistance to every move you make. The water offers 12-14% more resistance than when you exercise on land. Resistance does not allow for sudden body movements.

3. **Cooling Effect:** Water disperses heat more efficiently, so there is less chance of overheating. The water continuously cools the body. Exercise in the water is cooler and more comfortable than it is on land.

Options for exercising in the water include:

- Water Walking (See *Water Walking* in *Part I* of this manual for more information on starting a water walking program.)

- Water Aerobics

- Water Toning/Strength Training

- Flexibility Training

- Water Therapy and Rehabilitation

- Water Yoga and Relaxation

- Deep Water Exercise

- Deep Water Running

- Wall Exercises (deep or shallow)

- Water Fitness Products

- Lap Swimming

Brochures available from the USWFA:

- *Water Walking*

- *Water Exercise Promoter*

- *Doctor's Folder* (explanation of water walking)

Videos available from the USWFA:

- *Water Walking* – Learn the step (forward, backward, side) plus other helpful information.

- *Your Back Yard Swimming Pool Is Your Home Fitness Center* – Shows and explains a wide variety of exercise that can be done in any pool.

- *Deep Water Exercise* – Shows above and below shots of various methods of exercising in deep water.

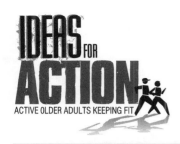

IDEAS FOR ACTION
ACTIVE OLDER ADULTS KEEPING FIT

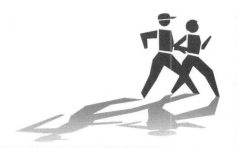

About the Editor and the Sporting Goods Manufacturers Association

Fitness consultant **Lynn Allen** is the president of Heartland Fitness in Lawrence, Kansas. Lynn works as a clinician and instructor on behalf of the President's Council on Physical Fitness and Sports and as an advisor to the Fitness Products Council of the Sporting Goods Manufacturers Association.

Lynn developed the Universal Fitness Institute (a four-day fitness certification course) for Universal Gym Equipment and has conducted the course throughout the United States, Europe, Australia, and the Pacific Rim. In addition, she has conducted fitness clinics for the U.S. military, the Australian military, and the Singapore Army. In 1993, Lynn designed an exercise room in the White House for President and Mrs. Clinton and developed personal exercise programs for each of them.

Lynn earned her bachelor's degree in recreational education with emphasis in

corporate fitness from the University of Iowa in 1981. She lives in Lawrence with her husband Terry and their children Angela and Chase.

The **Sporting Goods Manufacturers Association** (SGMA) comprises 14 nonprofit associations, councils, and committees that share a common goal of preserving and advancing recreational sports in the United States. Founded in 1906, the SGMA works to increase amateur sports participation.

The SGMA owns the Super Show, the world's largest trade show of sporting goods, equipment, apparel, and accessories. Proceeds from the Super Show support a host of national and local nonprofit sports organizations and programs. These funds are also used to sponsor many surveys and educational initiatives to benefit recreational sports.

Related Books from Human Kinetics

Exercise for Older Adults
ACE's Guide for Fitness Professionals
Richard T. Cotton, Editor, and Christine J. Ekeroth, Associate Editor
American Council on Exercise
Foreword by Sheryl Marks Brown
1998 • Paperback • 244 pp • Item BACE0942
ISBN 0-88011-942-X • $25.00 ($37.50 Canadian)

Developed under the leadership of the American Council on Exercise, this practical manual shows how to provide safe and effective exercise instruction for older adults. *Exercise for Older Adults* also clarifies the unique social and emotional implications that characterize this population. The authors provide valuable techniques and tools to help you motivate and communicate with older adults.

Exercise Programming for Older Adults
Kay A. Van Norman, MS
1995 • Paperback • 120 pp • Item BVAN0657
ISBN 0-87322-657-7 • $23.00 ($34.50 Canadian)

Exercise Programming for Older Adults explains how to develop, market, and manage a safe, effective fitness program for older adults. It covers many considerations unique to programming for seniors, such as physical conditions that can affect the safety of exercise and the ways psychological and social aspects of aging are influenced by exercise.

Physical Dimensions of Aging
Waneen W. Spirduso, EdD
Foreword by James E. Birren, PhD
1995 • Hardback • 448 pp • Item BSPI0323
ISBN 0-87322-323-3 • $55.00 ($82.50 Canadian)

Physical Dimensions of Aging is a landmark reference that provides the most comprehensive integration of research literature on physical aging available today. Waneen Spirduso, a renowned scholar in gerontology and kinesiology, has superbly translated dry facts into a well-written, easy-to-read text ideal for the increasing number of upper-division undergraduate and graduate courses on this topic.

Aging, Physical Activity, and Health
Roy J. Shephard, MD, PhD, DPE
1997 • Hardback • 496 pp • Item BSHE0889
ISBN 0-87322-889-8 • $45.00 ($67.50 Canadian)

Incorporating the latest theories on how aging and exercise affect a variety of medical conditions, author Roy J. Shephard provides conclusive physiological evidence that exercise reduces the risk of many diseases, maximizes independence, and improves the quality of life for the elderly. He also discusses the economic and social consequences of an aging society.

To request more information or to order, U.S. customers call 1-800-747-4457, e-mail us at humank@hkusa.com, or visit our website at www.humankinetics.com. Persons outside the U.S. can contact us via our website or use the appropriate telephone number, postal address, or e-mail address shown in the front of this book.

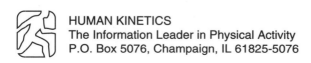
HUMAN KINETICS
The Information Leader in Physical Activity
P.O. Box 5076, Champaign, IL 61825-5076